ACADEMY OF NUTRITION AND DIETETICS
POCKET GUIDE TO

SECOND EDITION

Pediatric Nutrition Practice Group

Editors

Sharon Groh-Wargo, PhD, RD, LD

Melody Thompson, MS, RD, LD

Janice Hovasi Cox, MS, RD, CSP

eat right. Academy of Nutrition and Dietetics

ISBN: 978-0-88091-487-1

10 9 8 7 6 5 4 3 2

For more information on the Academy of Nutrition and Dietetics, visit: www.eatright.org

Contents

Continuing Professional Education

To access the Continuing Professional Education assessment that accompanies your purchase of this book, visit: https://publications.webauthor.com/go/form/form.cfm?xm_form_id=579

Contributors

Susan J. Carlson, MMSc, RDN, CSP, LD, CNSC
University of Iowa Children's Hospital
Iowa City, IA

Janice Hovasi Cox, MS, RD, CSP
The Children's Hospital at Bronson
Kalamazoo, MI

Marsha Dumm, MS, RD, LD
Nationwide Children's Hospital NICU at Riverside Methodist Hospital
Columbus, OH

Amy Gates, RD, CSP, LD
Georgia Regents University
Evans, GA

Sharon Groh-Wargo, PhD, RD, LD
MetroHealth Medical Center and
Case Western Reserve University
Cleveland, OH

Michelle Johnson, RD, CSP, LD
Abbott Nutrition Pediatric Scientific & Medical Affairs
Columbus, OH

Amy Jones, MS, RD, LD, CLC
Nationwide Children's Hospital
Columbus, OH

Anne M. Kavars, MS, RDN, LD, CNSC
University of Iowa Children's Hospital
Iowa City, IA

Ann E. Lewis, RD
St. Joseph's Hospital
Denver, CO

Allison Prince, MS, RDN, LD
Rainbow Babies and Children's Hospital
Cleveland, OH

Hunter Rametta, MS, RDN, LDN, CNSC
Brigham and Women's Hospital
Boston, MA

Amy Sapsford, RD, CSP, LD, CNSC
Cincinnati Children's Hospital Medical Center
Cincinnati, OH

Carrie Smith, MS, RD, LD
Cincinnati Children's Hospital Medical Center
Cincinnati, OH

Laurie J. Benson Szekely, MS, RD, LD
Akron Children's Hospital
Akron, OH

Melody Thompson, MS, RD, LD
Abbott Nutrition Pediatric Scientific & Medical Affairs, Nationwide Children's Hospital and The Ohio State University
Columbus, OH

Emily Trumpower, RD, CSP, CNSC
Mott Children's Hospital
Ann Arbor, MI

Reviewers

Meg Begany, RD, CSP, LDN, CNSC
The Children's Hospital of Philadelphia
Philadelphia, PA

Anne K. DeVitto, MS, RD, CSP
Sparrow Health System
Lansing, MI

Maria C. Hetherton, RD, CSP
UCSF Benioff Children's Hospital
San Francisco, CA

Laura Meredith-Dennis, RD
Dignity Health
Sacramento, CA

Patti H. Perks, MS, RD, CNSC
The University of Virginia Children's Hospital
Charlottesville, VA

Reviewers

Neonatal Terminology and Abbreviations

TERMINOLOGY

Neonate: newborn, birth to 28 days but sometimes used for a longer period of time

Neonatal: occurring during the first 28 days of life or very early infancy

Infancy: occurring during the first year of life

Low birth weight (LBW): < 2500 grams (5 pounds, 8 ounces)

Very low birth weight (VLBW): < 1500 grams (3 pounds, 5 ounces)

Extremely low birth weight (ELBW): < 1000 grams (2 pounds, 3 ounces)

Preterm (premature): gestational age (GA) < 37 weeks

Late preterm: GA ≥ 34 to < 37 weeks

Term: GA 37 to 42 weeks

Postterm: GA > 42 weeks

Small for gestational age (SGA): < 10th percentile birth weight for GA

Appropriate for gestational age (AGA): 10th to 90th percentile birth weight for GA

Large for gestational age (LGA): > 90th percentile birth weight for GA

ABBREVIATIONS

A/B/D: apnea, bradycardia, desaturations

AGA: appropriate for gestational age

ATN: acute tubular necrosis

BF: breastfeed or breastfeeding

BPD: bronchopulmonary dysplasia

CDH: congenital diaphragmatic hernia

CHD: congenital heart disease

CLD: chronic lung disease

CMV: cytomegalovirus

CPAP: continuous positive airway pressure

DBM/DHM/DM: donor breast milk/donor human milk/donor milk

DIC: disseminated intravascular coagulation

EBM: expressed breast milk

ECMO: extracorporeal membrane oxygenation

ELBW: extremely low birth weight

EN: enteral nutrition

EUGR: extrauterine growth restriction

FAS: fetal alcohol syndrome

FTT: failure to thrive

GA: gestational age

GIR: glucose infusion rate

$G_xP_xAb_xLC_x$: shorthand for gravida/para/abortion/living children (subscripts represent numbers of each)

HIE: hypoxic ischemic encephalopathy

HMF: human milk fortifier

IDM: infant of diabetic mother

IFE/IVFE: intravenous fat emulsion

IM: intramuscular

I&O: intake and output

IUGR: intrauterine growth restriction

IV: intravenous

IVH: intraventricular hemorrhage

KUB: kidneys, ureter, bladder (x-ray view)

LBW: low birth weight

LGA: large for gestational age

LOS: length of stay or late onset sepsis

LPI/LPTI: late preterm infant

MBM/MOM: mother's/maternal breast milk or own milk

MCT: medium-chain triglycerides

MEN: minimal enteral nutrition (also called priming, trophic and hypocaloric feeding, or gut stimulation)

mL/mm: milliliter/millimeter

NAS: neonatal abstinence syndrome

NEC: necrotizing enterocolitis

NG: nasogastric

NICU: neonatal intensive care unit

OFC: occipital frontal circumference (head circumference)

OG: orogastric

PDA: patent ductus arteriosus

PICC: percutaneous inserted central catheter

PN: parenteral nutrition

PNALD: parenteral nutrition-associated liver disease

PPHN: persistent pulmonary hypertension

PROM: premature rupture of membranes

PT: preterm

PVL: periventricular leukomalacia

RDS: respiratory distress syndrome

ROP: retinopathy of prematurity

RSV: respiratory syncytial virus

SBS: short bowel syndrome

SGA: small for gestational age

SIP: spontaneous intestinal perforation

SVD: spontaneous vaginal delivery

TEF/EA: tracheoesophageal fistula/esophageal atresia

TPN: total parenteral nutrition

TTN: transient tachypnea of the newborn

UAC: umbilical arterial catheter

UVC: umbilical venous catheter

VLBW: very low birth weight

Chapter 1

Nutrition Assessment

Laura J. Szekely, MS, RD, LD and
Melody Thompson, MS, RD, LD

OBJECTIVES

- List the components of infant nutrition assessment.
- Discuss anthropometric assessment and growth expectations.
- Review components of biochemical, clinical, and intake assessments.

INTRODUCTION

Nutrition assessment in infants includes the same components evaluated in other populations:

- Anthropometric assessment
- Biochemical assessment
- Clinical assessment
- Dietary intake assessment (parenteral, enteral, and oral)

Additionally, infant nutrition assessment includes classification of gestational age and size for gestational age.

A nutrition screen—often completed by a neonatal intensive care unit (NICU) nurse or dietetic technician, registered (DTR)—may be used to focus registered dietitian nutritionist (RDN) resources. Screening should be completed within 24 hours of admission (1,2). See Table 1.1 for an example of screening criteria (3). An RDN then completes an assessment on infants meeting designated criteria.

Table 1.1 Ohio Neonatal Nutritionists Screening Criteria for Identifying Hospitalized Infants at Highest Nutritional Risk

< 1 week of age a) > 15% weight loss from birth weight b) < 1 kg at birth
1–2 weeks of age a) < 70 kcal/kg/d b) Any continued weight loss
> 2 weeks of age a) Intake < 80% expected energy requirement < 70 kcal/kg/d (all IV) < 85 kcal/kg/d (IV/enteral) < 100 kcal/kg/d (all enteral) b) < 15 g/kg/d weight gain (< 36 weeks' gestational age) or < ½ expected g/d weight gain (> 36 weeks' gestational age) c) Prealbumin[a] < 8.0 mg/dL, or albumin < 2.5 g/dL BUN < 7 mg/dL Direct bilirubin > 2.0 mg/dL Serum phosphorus < 4 mg/dL Alkaline phosphatase > 600 U/L
> 2 months of age Any of the above for > 2 weeks of age plus: a) No source of dietary iron b) Continued total parenteral nutrition
Any infant with newly diagnosed NEC, BPD, cholestasis, osteopenia, cardiac disorders, neurologic problems, GI surgical anomalies, or metabolic aberrations

(continued)

Table 1.1 (continued)

Any infant with birth weight < 1.5 kg (and current weight < 2 kg) on full feedings but not receiving fortified human milk or preterm formula Abbreviations: BUN, blood urea nitrogen; NEC, necrotizing enterocolitis; BPD, bronchopulmonary dysplasia; GI, gastrointestinal.

[a]Include as criteria only if screening can be done in some time-efficient manner for entire unit; use values only as guide—compare to institutional normal ranges; while not reliable during inflammatory states, may indicate the infant with increased nutritional needs.

Source: Adapted from reference 3, Thompson M. Establishing and developing the position of the neonatal nutritionist. In: Groh-Wargo S, Thompson M, Cox JH, eds. *Nutritional Care for High-Risk Newborns.* Chicago, IL: Precept Press; 2000:605. Used with permission of the editors.

NEWBORN CLASSIFICATION OF GESTATIONAL AGE AND BIRTH WEIGHT

Newborn infant maturity and intrauterine growth are classified by gestational age, birth weight, and weight-for-gestational age.

- Gestational age can be estimated by maternal dates and by early (first/early second trimester) ultrasound exam (if available). The gestational age is also determined in the NICU by examining the infant's physical and neurological development on a reliable standardized instrument called the New Ballard score (available at www.ballardscore.com/files/ballardscore_scoresheet.pdf) (4). The gestational age classifies the infant as preterm, term, or postterm.
- The infant's birth weight is used to categorize the infant as (*a*) normal weight, (*b*) low birth weight (LBW), (*c*) very low birth weight (VLBW), or

(*d*) extremely low birth weight (ELBW). For specific definitions of LBW, VLBW, and ELBW, refer to Terms and Abbreviations.

- The infant's weight is plotted on an intrauterine growth chart to determine size for length of gestation—defined as (*a*) small for gestational age (SGA), (*b*) appropriate for gestational age (AGA), or (*c*) large for gestational age (LGA). For specific definitions of SGA, AGA, and LGA, refer to Terms and Abbreviations. In addition, infants may also be classified as intrauterine growth restricted (IUGR). Of note, although SGA and IUGR appear interchangeable, there is in fact a distinct difference. IUGR refers to the failure of the fetus to achieve normal predicted growth in utero (estimated fetal weight below the 10th percentile). SGA refers to a newborn with actual birth weight below the 10th percentile for gestational age (5). Finally, the term extrauterine growth restriction (EUGR) is a classification used to apply to infants who, although born with adequate intrauterine growth, fall below population norms during their hospitalization (weight < 10th percentile for corrected gestational age at the time of hospital discharge) (6).
- These classifications can help to guide or anticipate clinical care needs. For example, babies who are postterm and/or SGA or LGA are more likely to have hypoglycemia, polycythemia, birth asphyxia, and specific syndromes/anomalies than are term AGA babies. Prematurity is also associated with a host of potential morbidities—many of which are discussed in this pocket guide.

ANTHROPOMETRIC ASSESSMENT

Postnatal growth—with consistent and comprehensive monitoring—is an important health care outcome measure for high-risk infants (7). Anthropometric measurements are rapid, inexpensive, and noninvasive to obtain.

Measurement of body weight, length, and head circumference is the predominant method used to monitor infant growth, detect growth abnormalities, and assess nutritional status in infants. Measurements are plotted on percentile growth curves for comparison against established reference data. Serial measures of growth are compulsory in assessing response to nutrition support in hospitalized infants. Satisfactory postnatal growth is associated with shortened lengths of hospitalization and improved cognitive development (8–11).

Weight

Method

The nude infant is weighed on a regularly calibrated digital gram scale.

Uses and Interpretation

- Body weight comprises the total mass of the infant's lean tissue, fat, and extracellular and intracellular fluid compartments.
- As gestational age increases, extracellular fluid volume decreases and lean tissue and fat mass increase.
- Initial postnatal weight loss is attributed to contraction of body water compartments and catabolism of endogenous stores before energy and nutrient needs are met (8).

- Expected initial postnatal weight loss ranges between 8% and 15%, with greater loss found in the smallest, most immature infants (12).
- Initial weight loss reaches its nadir by approximately 4 to 6 days of life (8).
- Birth weight is optimally regained by 2 weeks with the extremely premature infant; the very ill infant sometimes requires 3 weeks (8,9,13).
- Daily body weights allow assessment of fluid status.
- Expected incremental weight gain in LBW infants changes over time, with advancing gestational age. In general, a growth velocity (GV) goal of 15 to 20 g/kg/d is often used for LBW infants. If desired, specific GV goals can be calculated from intrauterine growth charts over various time intervals at specific percentiles. A multicenter cohort study of ELBW infants showed that, once birth weight was regained, weight gain of >18 g/kg/d was associated with better neurodevelopmental and growth outcomes than those seen with lower growth velocities (10).
- Actual GV over time can be calculated for an individual infant. Calculating GV using an exponential method is the most accurate of five methods tested and has been validated in ELBW infants (14,15). A limitation of this method is that it requires computerized calculations. A method that is close in accuracy to the exponential method can be calculated using the following equation (14):

$$GV\ (g/kg/d) = \frac{[1000 \times (W_n - W_1)]}{\{(D_n - D_1) \times [(W_n + W_1)/2]\}}$$

Where W = weight in grams, D = day, 1 = beginning of time interval chosen and n = the end of that time interval in days.

For example, here is how to calculate GV for an infant who weighs 1,100 g on day 12 and 1,400 g on day 26:

$$GV = \frac{[1000 \times (1440 - 1100)]}{\{(26 - 12) \times [(1440 + 1100/2]\}}$$

$$GV = \frac{[1000 \times 340]}{\{14 \times 1270\}}$$

$$GV = \frac{340{,}000}{17{,}780}$$

$$GV = 19.1 \text{ g/kg/d}$$

This equation, which uses average weight in the denominator, is more accurate than methods using birth weight or other weights in the denominator (14).

Limitations

Weight gain does not accurately reflect lean body mass changes, especially when edema or dehydration is present (8,9).

Length

Method

Ideally, two people are required to obtain an accurate linear measurement using an infant length board. One person holds the infant's head against the fixed headboard; the other measurer gently flattens the infant's knees and guides the footboard toward the infant's flat feet. In some clinical settings, however, infant length is *estimated* using a tape measure, sacrificing accuracy for expediency.

Uses and Interpretation

- Weekly length measurements have the following advantages over the measurement of weight (16):
  - Length more accurately reflects lean tissue mass.
  - Length is not influenced by fluid status.
  - Length is a better indicator of long-term growth.
- Expected incremental gain in crown-heel length in LBW infants is ≥ 0.9 cm/week (8,9,17).

Limitations

Length is often more difficult to accurately determine—requiring a length board and two measurers—than either weight or head circumference (8,9).

Head Circumference

Method

The largest occipital frontal circumference (OFC), commonly referred to as head circumference (HC) is measured with a flexible tape measure.

Uses and Interpretation

- During the first postnatal week, HC may decrease by approximately 0.5 cm due to extracellular fluid space contraction (8).
- Head circumference is monitored weekly; mean weekly gain in LBW infants is ≥ 0.9 cm/week (8,9,17).
- More frequent assessment may be indicated for infants with micro- or macrocephaly or with suspected abnormal increases in head circumference (> 1.25 cm/week) (8).

Limitations

Cerebral edema, hydrocephalus, compression due to the administration device for nasal continuous positive airway pressure (NCPAP), or the addition or removal of external apparatus may interfere with accuracy of head circumference measurements.

Weight-for-Length

Method

Using the growth chart, ideal weight-for-length is identified by finding the weight that is approximately on the same percentile as the infant's length measurement percentile.

Uses and Interpretation

- Determining ideal weight-for-length is helpful in assessing symmetry of growth.
- Current weight expressed as a percentage of ideal weight-for-length can be used to identify infants at risk for under- or overnutrition (8). This measurement should be used with caution and optimally when the length measurement is known to be accurate.

Regional Anthropometry

Regional anthropometry is not routinely assessed. (It is used primarily in research settings.)

Uses and Interpretation

- Triceps skinfold (TSF) and midarm circumference, or the ratios and formulas derived from these measurements, are reported to be good predictors of infant body composition, growth, and metabolic complications for infants who are overgrown or undergrown during gestation (16).

- Standards are available for infants between 24 and 41 weeks' gestation and can be used to compare measurements of an individual infant to reference values or to assess individual changes over time (8). Of note, this measurement may be most helpful in patients with compromised conditions such as ascites, conjoined twins, and chronic ventilator dependency.

Limitations

- Examiner measurement technique variability, as well as critical illness, hydration status, and positioning of infants, can make these measurements invalid or unreliable (8).
- The use of calipers to measure TSF may not be feasible in extremely immature infants who have delicate, easily punctured skin.
- Weight, length, and head circumference have been found to be the most reliable measurements and are highly predictive of both fat and lean mass (8).

Growth Charts

Growth charts provide the basis for growth and nutrition assessment of high-risk infants by presenting a comparison of an infant's actual size and growth trajectory to reference data (8,9).

Two types of charts are presently available for growth assessment:

- Charts developed using intrauterine growth data
- Charts developed using postnatal growth data

In most NICUs, the infant's measurements are plotted sequentially and electronically and may be accessed utilizing both intrauterine and postnatal growth charts via the electronic health record as available.

Intrauterine Growth Charts

Intrauterine growth charts are based on a compilation of cross-sectional measurements of birth weight, length, and head circumference from infants of varying gestational ages at birth (8,9). They represent fetal growth and are presented as the goal for preterm infant growth (8,9). The infant's weight, length, and head circumference can be plotted weekly on these curves.

Gender-specific intrauterine growth charts based on precise measurements of gestational age have been developed and revised to reflect recommended growth goals for preterm infants (the fetus, followed by the term infant) and support an improved transition of preterm infant growth to the World Health Organization (WHO) growth charts (see Figures 1.1 and 1.2) (17). A free copy of the development article for the 2013 Fenton growth charts can be found online at www.biomedcentral.com/1471-2431/13/59.

Figure 1.1 2013 Preterm Growth Chart for Girls

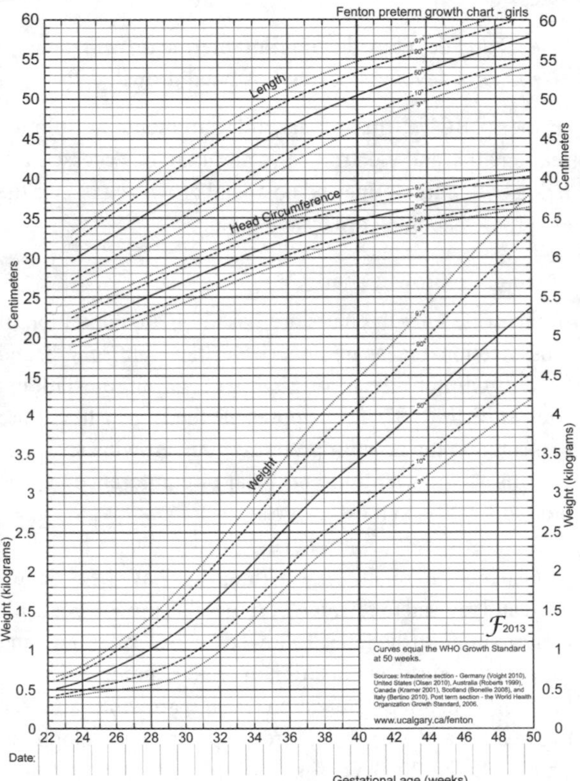

Source: Reprinted with permission from reference 17, Fenton TR. A systematic review and meta-analysis to revise the Fenton growth chart for preterm infants. *BMC Pediatr*. 2013; 13:5914. A downloadable version of this chart is available at http://ucalgary.ca/fenton/files/fenton/fenton2013growthchartgirls.pdf.

Figure 1.2 2013 Preterm Growth Chart for Boys

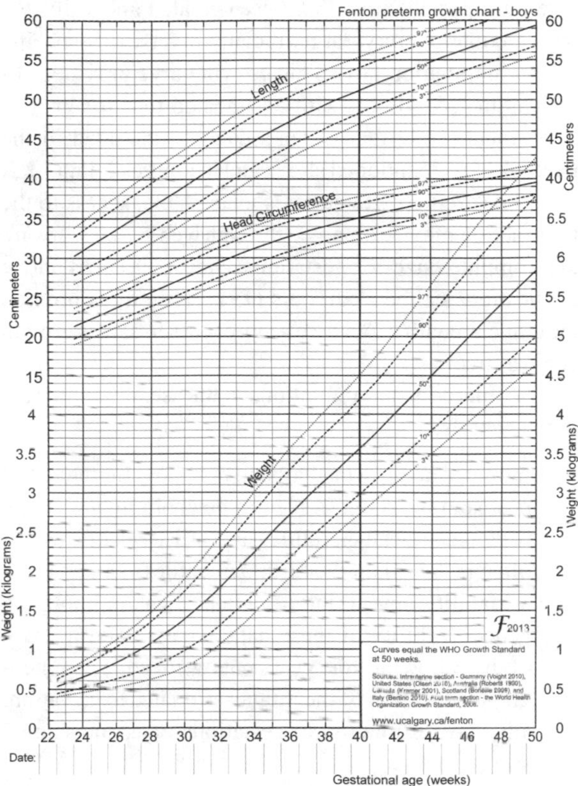

Source: Reprinted with permission from reference 17, Fenton TR. A systematic review and meta-analysis to revise the Fenton growth chart for preterm infants. *BMC Pediatr*. 2013; 13:5914. A downloadable version of this chart is available at http://ucalgary.ca/fenton/files/fenton/fenton2013growthchartboys.pdf.

In addition, some NICUs may choose to utilize an alternate intrauterine curve that Olsen created and validated with a contemporary, large, racially diverse US-specific sample population (18). This growth curve provides clinicians in US NICUs with an updated tool for growth assessment. Note that Olsen's data are included in the Fenton charts mentioned above and in Figures 1.1 and 1.2.

If a desired growth curve is unavailable, access to the information may be obtained through web-based software that computes size-for-gestational age, or via smart phone applications called PediTools (19). These tools provide the clinician with a variety of approaches to assess growth comparatively.

The following are limitations to the use of intrauterine growth charts:

- Intrauterine growth charts do not allow for the initial postnatal weight loss seen in newborn infants; body weight and head circumference at 1 week of age will often be less than the birth percentiles (8).
- Variability among the intrauterine charts limits the generalizability of these data. Charts vary in terms of the following: the years data were collected, geographic location of the infants as related to elevation, ethnicity, estimation of gestational age, and sample size (8,9).
- Typically, the preterm infant's growth will parallel and not exceed the intrauterine growth curve of a fetus of similar gestational age (8,9).

Postnatal Growth Charts

Postnatal growth charts based on a large sample of infants (from a broad geographic area in the United States) receiving current neonatal care have been published (20). These charts provide a reference for expected weight, length, and head circumference changes starting at various birth weights. Because they were developed from postnatal growth data, they reflect the initial weight loss that occurs in infants during the first week of life (8,9).

The following are limitations to the use of postnatal growth charts:

- Postnatal growth charts do not show an infant's GV or "catch-up" growth relative to the fetus (8).
- Postnatal growth charts were likely influenced by the medical and nutritional support practices used for the sample infants (8).

The preterm infant's ideal growth pattern remains undefined. Studies are in process to determine prescriptive standards for fetal and preterm growth and may be available following the completion of the INTERGROWTH-21st Project (17,21).

Growth Assessment

Weight gain is used to identify infants with mean weight gains that are less than desired growth (< 15g/kg/d) or more than desired growth (> 35 g/d) during a week's period of time (9).

Infants at high risk of poor weight gain include those with extreme prematurity, chronic lung disease, severe intraventricular hemorrhage, necrotizing enterocolitis (NEC), and late-onset sepsis (8,9). Factors that may contribute to poor weight gain include the following (8,9):

- Insufficient fluid, energy, or nutrient intake
- Improper preparation of feeding
- Feeding intolerance
- Acidosis

- Hypoxia
- Anemia
- Chronic diuretic administration
- Temperature instability/cold stress

Factors that may contribute to excessive weight gain include the following (8,9):

- Excessive fluid, energy, or nutrient intake
- Improper preparation of feeding
- Chronic systemic steroid administration (in addition to excessive weight gain, this treatment may contribute to the loss of lean mass and decreased linear growth)

BIOCHEMICAL ASSESSMENT

Biochemical (laboratory) data can be useful markers of nutritional status. Specific laboratory tests may help detect nutritional deficiency or toxicity prior to the appearance of clinical symptoms.

Many factors, however, can alter serum levels and must be considered when interpreting laboratory results (8). These factors include:

- Storage and processing of the specimen
- Laboratory method used
- Technician accuracy
- Disease state or medical treatment, including blood transfusions
- Infant's state of hydration

It is important to note trends in laboratory results as well as the speed and direction of changes. Laboratory tests are interpreted with caution and used to complement other nutrition assessment data (8).

Parenteral Nutrition

Regular assessment of laboratory data is necessary for infants receiving parenteral nutrition (PN). Early detection of metabolic complications of PN is facilitated by analysis of electrolytes, blood urea nitrogen, creatinine, calcium, magnesium, phosphorus, glucose, liver enzymes, visceral proteins, and triglycerides.

Frequent monitoring may be required as PN solutions are initiated and adjusted to meet the specific energy and nutrient needs of individual infants. Once stable, laboratory monitoring every 7 to 14 days is sufficient (8). See Table 1.2 (8).

Table 1.2 Suggested Monitoring Schedule for Infants Receiving Parenteral Nutrition Support

	Initial Phase[a]	Stable Phase[b]
Growth:		
• Weight	• Daily	• Daily
• Length	• Baseline	• Weekly
• Head circumference	• Baseline	• Weekly
Intake and output	Daily	Daily
Glucose:		
• Serum	• As indicated	• As indicated
• Urine	• As indicated	• As indicated
Electrolytes	2–3 times/wk	Every 1–2 wks
Calcium, magnesium, phosphorus	2–3 times/wk	Every 1–2 wks
Triglycerides	Daily during dose increase	Every 1–2 wks
BUN/creatinine	2–3 times/wk	Every 1–2 wks
Serum proteins	Baseline	Every 2–3 wks

(continued)

Table 1.2 Suggested Monitoring Schedule for Infants Receiving Parenteral Nutrition Support (continued)

Liver enzymes—including direct bilirubin	Baseline	Every 2–3 wks
Alkaline phosphatase	Baseline	Every 2–3 wks
Blood cell count	Baseline	Every 2–3 wks
Vitamin and trace mineral status or other specific tests	As indicated	As indicated

Abbreviations: BUN, blood urea nitrogen.

[a]In the initial phase, parenteral nutrition solutions are adjusted to meet the specific energy and nutrient needs of individual infants. This period generally lasts for < 1 week for parenteral support.

[b]In the stable phase, the infant is in a metabolically steady state. For clinically stable infants receiving an adequate nutrient intake with desired growth, the interval between laboratory measurements may be increased beyond the above recommendations.

Source: Data are from reference 8.

Enteral Nutrition

Biochemical assessment of the infant receiving enteral nutrition (EN) is not well delineated. In medically unstable infants, it may be desirable to follow serial indicators of hematologic, protein, mineral, and electrolyte status. Routine laboratory monitoring, however, is not indicated for medically stable infants receiving enteral nutrition at advised levels and achieving adequate growth (8). See Table 1.3 (8).

Table 1.3 Suggested Monitoring for Infants Receiving Enteral Nutrition Support

	Interval
Growth: • Weight • Length • Head circumference	 • Daily • Weekly • Weekly
Intake and output	Daily
	Indication
Electrolytes	Diuretics; renal disease
BUN and creatinine	Renal disease
BUN alone	Protein intake adjustment
Phosphorus, alkaline phosphatase, 25 (OH) vitamin D	Osteopenia screen
Albumin, prealbumin	Poor nutrition history, slow growth, edema
Liver enzymes including direct bilirubin	Cholestasis
Blood cell count	Anemia
Vitamin and trace mineral status or other specific tests	As indicated

Abbreviations: BUN, blood urea nitrogen.
Source: Data are from reference 8.

Limitations of Biochemical Assessment

High-risk infants cannot afford to lose much blood volume for biochemical tests. The laboratory performing the tests for small preterm infants must be capable of using techniques that require only microliters of blood (8).

The cost, relative usefulness, and turnaround time of a complex laboratory test should be considered before the test is done (8). Proposed laboratory monitoring protocols for infants receiving PN or enterally fed infants with chronic illness, such as chronic lung disease, or poor growth are provided in Tables 1.2 and 1.3 (8).

Although it is best to use the individual laboratory's reference ranges, Table 1.4 gives rounded average ranges of normal laboratory values for infants beyond the first week of life (22–24).

Table 1.4 Normal Laboratory Values for Term and Preterm Infants

Test	Normal Range[a]
Glucose	50–100 mg/dL
Electrolytes • Sodium • Potassium • Chloride	 • 130–145 mEq/L • 3.5–6 mEq/L • 100–110 mEq/L
Calcium	6–12 mg/dL
Magnesium	1.5–2.5 mg/dL
Phosphorus	5–9 mg/dL
Triglycerides	< 200 mg/dL
BUN	7–20 mg/dL
Creatinine	0.2–1 mg/dL
Albumin	3–5 g/dL
Prealbumin	10–25 mg/dL
Direct bilirubin	< 0.2 mg/dL
Alkaline phosphatase	100–500 U/L
Hemoglobin	10–15 g/dL
Hematocrit	30%–45%

Abbreviation: BUN, blood urea nitrogen.

[a]Rounded average ranges to use beyond the first week of life.

Source: Data are from references 22–24. Table is used by permission of Melody Thompson.

CLINICAL ASSESSMENT

Clinical assessment includes observation of the infant's general condition, bedside nursing documentation, feeding tolerance, and medical status. Of note, the Nutrition Focused Physical Assessment is an additional tool utilized in assessing nutritional status, but is an evolving practice and not yet refined in the neonatal population (25).

Apgar Scores

Apgar scores are recorded in the medical record. These scores are an assessment of a newborn's heart rate, respiratory effort, muscle tone, reflex irritability, and color. Scores are tallied at 1 and 5 minutes after birth and may be repeated every 5 minutes until the infant's condition stabilizes.

- Scores range from 0 to 10.
- Total scores of 0 to 3 indicate profound distress.
- Scores of 4 to 6 show moderate difficulty.
- Scores of 7 to 10 represent normal adaptation to extrauterine life.
- Low Apgar scores with no improvement may warrant a cautious approach to enteral feeding initiation and advancement.

Skin

Carefully observe the infant's skin (see Table 1.5) (22,26). Skin color is an important indicator of cardiorespiratory function. Additionally, notice any devices for respiratory, feeding, or excretory assistance that may influence feeding (such as ventilator tubing, nasal prongs, feeding tube, pacifier, urinary catheter, or ostomy).

Table 1.5 Infant Clinical Assessment: Skin

Observation	Possible Clinical Significance
Color	
Pallor (washed-out, whitish)	• Birth asphyxia • Shock (altered perfusion) • Anemia (iron and/or vitamin deficiency) • Chronic disease • Patent ductus arteriosus
Plethora (deep, rosy red)	• Polycythemia • Overoxygenated • Overheated
Jaundice	• Yellowish: indirect hyperbilirubinemia • Greenish: direct hyperbilirubinemia
Central cyanosis (bluish skin, tongue, lips)	• Low O_2 saturation, may be congenital heart disease or lung disease (concern about gut perfusion)
Acrocyanosis (bluish hands and feet only)	• Cold stress • Hypovolemia
Mottling (lacy red pattern)	• Normal variation • Cold stress • Hypovolemia • Sepsis
Fluid status	
Periorbital or generalized edema; bulging fontanel	• Overhydration • Protein deficiency
Dry mucous membranes; sunken fontanel; lack of tears; poor skin turgor	• Dehydration

(continued)

Table 1.5 Infant Clinical Assessment: Skin (continued)

Integrity	
Dermatitis	• EFA, B vitamin, or zinc deficiency
Flaky paint dermatitis	• Protein deficiency
Poor wound healing	• Zinc, vitamin C, calorie, or protein deficiency
Texture	
Scaly, dry	• EFA, vitamin A, or zinc deficiency
Excessive initial peeling	• Postterm: normal variant

Abbreviations: O_2, oxygen; EFA, essential fatty acid.
Source: Data are from references 22 and 26. Table is used by permission of Melody Thompson.

Vital Signs, Urine and Stool Output, and Feeding Tolerance

Review the infant's vital signs and urine and stool output (see Tables 1.6, 1.7, and 1.8) (22,24,26). An infant's first urine output is within 24 hours of birth; first stool is within 24 to 48 hours of birth (24). Also note signs of feeding tolerance or intolerance (see bulleted list of feeding intolerance signs in Chapter 3 on page 107).

Table 1.6 Infant Clinical Assessment: Vital Signs

Temperature

- Normal range: 36.5–37.5°C (97.7–99.5°F)
- Hypo- and hyperthermia associated with increased BMR, increased O_2 consumption, decreased weight gain

(continued)

Table 1.6 Infant Clinical Assessment: Vital Signs (continued)

Respiratory rate
- Normal range: 30–60 breaths/min[a]
- Tachypnea (> 60 breaths/min) is a contraindication for nipple feeding
- Apnea (absence of breathing for > 20 seconds) and/or bradycardia (see below) suggest cardiorespiratory instability: feed cautiously

Heart rate
- Normal range: 100–180 beats/min[a]
- Tachycardia (> 180 beats/min) associated with increased energy consumption
- Bradycardia (< 100 beats/min) (see apnea above)

Abbreviations: BMR, basal metabolic rate; O_2, oxygen.

[a]Respiratory rate and heart rate may be lower when sleeping; higher when crying.

Source: Data are from references 22 and 26. Table is used by permission of Melody Thompson.

Table 1.7 Infant Clinical Assessment: Urine Output

Urine volume
- Normal range: 1–3 mL/kg/h *or* 5–7 mL/kg/h with diuresis
- < 1 mL/kg/h = oliguria
- No urine output = anuria
- If the infant is oliguric or anuric, consider reducing volume and PRSL of feeding for conservative treatment of ARF

Urine-specific gravity
- Normal range: 1.001–1.020
- > 1.020 may be associated with dehydration, increased feeding concentration, increased PRSL, or decreased fluid intake

Urine-reducing substances
- Normal finding: negative
- Glucosuria associated with IV glucose load above renal threshold; or rule out galactosemia

Abbreviations: PRSL, potential renal solute load; ARF, acute renal failure.

Source: Data are from reference 22. Table is used by permission of Melody Thompson.

Table 1.8 Infant Clinical Assessment: Stool Output

Timing of first stool
- Normal range: Within 48 hours of birth
- No stool: consider bowel obstruction, imperforate anus, aganglionosis, Hirschsprung's disease

Frequency (when enteral feedings are established)
- Normal range: From every feeding to every 3 days
- Excessive watery stools: evaluate hydration status
- Infrequent stools: consider strictures

Color
- Normal range: Initially: tarry, dark (meconium); later: yellow to green to brown
- Black stools: may be associated with occult blood
- Clay-colored stools: may indicate cholestasis or decreased bile flow

Blood
- Normal: None present
- Blood present: early, consider swallowed maternal blood; later, consider anal fissure, enteral tube trauma, gastritis/stress ulcer, feeding intolerance (protein allergy), colitis, or necrotizing enterocolitis

pH
- Normal range: 5–7
- < 5 suggestive of carbohydrate malabsorption (colonic bacterial fermentation produces short-chain fatty acids, which lower stool pH)

Reducing substances
- Normal: None after first week of life
- Unabsorbed sugars (> ¼%) suggest carbohydrate malabsorption

Source: Data are from references 22, 24, and 26. Table is used by permission of Melody Thompson.

Medical Records

A review of interdisciplinary care could include reviewing the medical record, as well as participating and listening on rounds for the following:

- Potential drug-nutrient interactions
- Radiology reports—noting studies relevant to gastrointestinal (GI) anatomy and function (eg, upper gastrointestinal [UGI], barium enema, abdominal ultrasound, etc) and noting any evidence of osteopenia (See Chapter 15.)
- Neurology reports—noting any evidence of neurologic problems (See Chapter 13.)
- Maternal history of relevance: intent to breastfeed, weight gain during pregnancy, illnesses (including gestational diabetes; surgeries [breast implants/reduction, gastric bypass]; deficiencies [vitamin D]; family history of food allergies; and use of alcohol or drugs)

DIETARY INTAKE ASSESSMENT

Data Collection

To assess dietary intake, review the medical record or nursing flow sheets to determine nutrient sources—PN, IV solutions, human milk, human milk fortifier (HMF), infant formula, and vitamin, mineral, or other modular supplements.

Data Analysis

The dietary intake assessment should include both qualitative and quantitative analyses:

- In the qualitative analysis, consider whether current nutrient solutions are appropriate for the patient's gestational age, size, tolerance issues (if any), and diagnoses.
- In the quantitative analysis, calculate nutrient intakes (at least mL/kg/d, kcal/kg/d, and protein g/kg/d).
    - PN calculations (including dextrose, crystalline amino acids, and IV fat g/kg/d) are done in the same way for infants as they are for other populations.
    - Additionally, fluid, dextrose, and/or electrolytes in IV drip medications often contribute substantially to an infant's nutrient intake and are calculated.
    - Occasionally, even medication flushes influence the small infant's glucose or electrolyte status.
    - A more detailed targeted nutrient intake analysis may be done on intakes of infants with certain diagnoses or conditions (eg, assessing calcium, phosphorus, and vitamin D intakes for infants with osteopenia).

Calculations of nutrient intakes are compared with recommended intakes (see Chapters 2 and 3 for PN and EN recommendations) and interpreted in light of the infant's medical condition and growth. See Box 1.1 for an example of how to calculate nutrient intake.

Box 1.1 Sample Nutrient Intake Calculation for 1,500-g Preterm Infant

Intake

Maternal milk fortified to 24 kcal/fl oz with human milk fortifier; taking 28 mL every 3 hours

Calculations

28 mL × 8 feedings/d = 224 mL/d ÷ 1.5 kg = 149 mL/kg/d

149 mL/kg/d × 0.8 kcal/mL[a] = 119 kcal/kg/d

149 mL/kg/d × 0.028 g protein/mL[a] = 4.2 g protein/kg/d

[a]For most precise calculations, consult the specific manufacturer's literature.

SUMMARY

Screening should be completed within 24 hours of NICU admission (see Table 1.1). An RDN then completes an assessment on designated infants. This assessment should include all of the following:

- **Anthropometric assessment:** Obtain accurate measurements of weight, length, and head circumference. Plot on appropriate growth curves. Consider infant's classification (ie, gestational age, birth weight, and weight for gestational age). Interpret/analyze growth pattern or trend.
- **Biochemical assessment:** Review appropriate biochemical data. Interpret in light of patient's condition.
- **Clinical assessment:** Look at the patient and medical record; make clinical observations.
- **Dietary intake assessment:** Evaluate intake to assess what and how much is administered. Calculate intake—at least fluids, energy, and protein, all per kilogram per day.

All components of nutrition assessment (anthropometric, biochemical, clinical, and dietary intake assessments with infant classification) are used to develop the infant's nutrition care plan and form the basis for documentation in the medical record.

REFERENCES

1. The Joint Commission. *Comprehensive Accreditation Manual for Hospitals (CAMH)*. Oakbrook Terrace, IL: Joint Commission on Accreditation of Healthcare Organizations; 2015.
2. Corkins MR, Griggs KC, Groh-Wargo S, Han-Markey TL, Helms RA, Muir LV, Szeszycki EE. Task Force on Standards for Nutrition Support: Pediatric Hospitalized Patients; and the American Society for Parenteral and Enteral Nutrition Board of Directors. Standards for nutrition support: pediatric hospitalized patients. *Nutr Clin Pract.* 2013;28:263–276.
3. Thompson M. Establishing and developing the position of neonatal nutritionist. In: Groh-Wargo S, Thompson M, Cox JH, eds. *Nutritional Care for High-Risk Newborns.* Chicago, IL: Precept Press; 2000:605.
4. Ballard JL, Khoury JC, Wedig K, Wang L, Eilers-Walsman BL, Lipp R. New Ballard score, expanded to include extremely premature infants. *J Pediatr*. 1991;119:417–423.
5. Chauhan SP, Gupta LM, Hendrix NW, Berghella V. Intrauterine growth restriction: comparison of American College of Obstetricians and Gynecologists practice bulletin with other national guidelines. *Am J Obstet Gynecol*. 2009;200:409.e1–409.e6.
6. Ruth VA. Extrauterine growth restriction: A review of the literature. *Neonatal Network*. 2008;27(3):177–184.
7. Kuzma-O'Reilly B, Duenas ML, Greecher C, Kimberlin L, Mjusce D, Miller D, Walker DJ. Evaluation, development, and implementation of potentially better practices in neonatal intensive care nutrition. *Pediatrics*. 2003;111(4 Pt 2):e46–e470.
8. Moyer-Mileur LJ. Anthropometry and laboratory assessment of very low birth weight infants: the most helpful measurements and why. *Semin Perinatol.* 2007;31:96–103.
9. Anderson DM. Nutritional assessment and therapeutic interventions for the preterm infant. *Clin Perinatol.* 2002;29:313–326.

10. Ehrenkranz RA, Dusick AM, Vohr BR, Wright LL, Wrage LA, Poole WK. National Institutes of Child Health and Human Development Neonatal Research Network. Growth in the neonatal intensive care unit influences neurodevelopmental and growth outcomes of extremely low birth weight infants. *Pediatrics*. 2006;117:1253–1261.
11. Ramel SE, Demerath EW, Gray HL, Younge N, Boys C, Georgieff MK. The relationship of poor linear growth velocity with neonatal illness and two-year neurodevelopment in preterm infants. *Neonatology.* 2012;102:19–24.
12. Bell EF, Acarregui MJ. Restricted versus liberal water intake for preventing morbidity and mortality in newborn infants. *Cochrane Database Syst Rev.* 2008 Jan 23;(1):CD000503.
13. Clark R, Olsen IE, Spitzer AR. Assessment of neonatal growth in prematurely born infants. *Clin Perinatol*. 2014;41:295–307.
14. Patel AL, Engstrom JL, Meier PP, Kimura RE. Accuracy of methods for calculating postnatal growth velocity for extremely low birth weight infants. *Pediatrics*. 2005;116(6):1466–1473.
15. Patel AL, Engstrom JL, Meier PP, Jegier BJ, Kimura RE. Calculating postnatal growth velocity in very low birth weight (VLBW) infants. *J Perinatol.* 2009;29:618–622.
16. Roche A, Sun S. *Human Growth: Assessment and Interpretation.* 1st ed. New York, NY: Cambridge University Press; 2003:1–9.
17. Fenton TR. A systematic review and meta-analysis to revise the Fenton growth chart for preterm infants. *BMC Pediatr*. 2013; 13:5914.
18. Olsen I. New intrauterine growth curves based on United States data. *Pediatrics*. 2010;125;e214–e224.
19. Peditools. www.peditools.org. Accessed November 26, 2014.
20. Ehrenkranz RA, Younes N, Lemons JA, Fanaroff AA, Donovan EF, Wright LL, Katsikiotis V, Tyson JE, Oh W, Shankaran S, Bauer CR, Korones SB, Stoll BJ, Stevenson DK, Papile L. Longitudinal growth of hospitalized very low birth weight infants. *Pediatrics*. 1999;104(2 Pt 1):280–289.
21. Villar J, Altman DG, Purwar M, Noble JA, Knight HE, Ruyan P, Cheikh Ismail L, Barros FC, Lambert A, Papageorghiou AT, Carvalho M, Jaffer YA, Bertino E, Gravett MG, Bhutta ZA, Kennedy SH; International Fetal and Newborn Growth Consortium for the 21st Century. The objectives, design and implementation of the INTERGROWTH-21st Project. *BJOG*. 2013;120 (Suppl 2):9–26.

22. Hockenberry MJ, Wilson D. *Wong's Nursing Care of Infants and Children.* 9th ed. St Louis, MO: Mosby Elsevier; 2011.
23. Gilbert-Barness E, Barness LA. *Clinical Use of Pediatric Diagnostic Tests*. 2nd ed. Washington, DC: IOS Press; 2010.
24. Martin RJ, Fanaroff AA, Walsh MC, eds. *Fanaroff and Martin's Neonatal-Perinatal Medicine: Diseases of the Fetus and Infant.* 9th ed. Philadelphia, PA: Mosby Elsevier; 2011.
25. Green Corkins K. Nutrition-focused physical examination in pediatric patients. *Nutr Clin Pract.* 2015(2);30:203–209.
26. Gomella TL, ed. *Neonatology: Management, Procedures, On-Call Problems, Diseases, and Drugs.* 7th ed. New York, NY: Lange Medical Books/McGraw-Hill; 2013.

Chapter 2

Parenteral Nutrition

Susan J. Carlson, MMSc, RDN, CSP, LD, CNSC, and
Anne Kavars, MS, RDN, LD, CNSC

OBJECTIVES

- Write a parenteral nutrition prescription for prematurely born neonate.
- List the parameters monitored to ensure safe and adequate parenteral delivery of nutrients.
- Describe modifications to standard parenteral nutrient delivery that may be needed to address typical clinical conditions encountered during the neonatal period, such as alterations in electrolyte or serum glucose levels, fluid status, mineral depletion, hypertriglyceridemia, or cholestasis.

INDICATIONS FOR USE

Parenteral nutrition (PN) is used during the neonatal period, initially to prevent negative energy and protein balance, and subsequently to support normal growth until adequate enteral feedings can be established. Indications for PN include the following (1,2):

- Prematurity—immature motility/function of the gastrointestinal (GI) tract. Most infants with gestational age (GA) at birth < 32 weeks or birth weight < 1,800 g and many infants with GA at birth < 35 weeks and/or birth weight < 2,200 g will benefit from supplemental PN as enteral feeds are typically advanced cautiously (eg, < 30 mL/kg/d).

- Necrotizing enterocolitis (NEC) or spontaneous intestinal perforation (SIP)
- Congenital GI anomalies requiring surgical repair and/or disorders of impaired GI motility (eg, gastroschisis, omphalocele, bowel obstruction, bowel atresia, Hirschsprung's disease, ileus from surgery or sepsis)
- Malabsorption syndromes (short bowel syndrome, cystic fibrosis with meconium ileus)
- Syndromes or medications associated with impaired GI perfusion (eg, congenital heart disease, patent ductus arteriosus [PDA], hypotension, hypoxic ischemic encephalopathy [HIE], nonsteroidal anti-inflammatory drugs [NSAIDs] such as indomethacin and ibuprofen)
- Chylothorax that is refractory to low long-chain triglyceride (LCT) enteral feedings
- Delayed initiation or advancement of enteral feeds

DURATION OF PN

Initiation of PN

- Weight < 1.5 kg: Initiate within 24 hours of life
- Weight 1.5 to 2.5 kg: Initiate within the first 1 to 2 days of life
- Weight > 2.5 kg or term GA: Initiate within the first 2 to 3 days of life

Termination of PN

PN should be continued until the infant tolerates enteral feedings at least 75% to 80% of energy goal or is within 2 to 3 days of achieving goal enteral volume.

NUTRIENT DOSE RECOMMENDATIONS

Table 2.1 summarizes PN dose recommendations for energy, macronutrients, electrolytes, and minerals (1–7). Recommendations for selected nutrients are also discussed in greater detail later in this chapter.

Table 2.1 Daily Parenteral Nutrition Dose Recommendations for Energy, Macronutrients, Electrolytes, and Minerals

Basal energy[a], kcal/kg/d • Initial dose: 35–50 • Transition dose: 35–50 • Growing premature infants: 46–55 • Growing term infants: 55
Total energy[b], kcal/kg/d • Initial dose: 35–50 • Transition dose: 60–85 • Growing premature infants: 90–115 • Growing term infants: 90–108
Dextrose[c], mg/kg/min • Initial dose: 5 • Transition dose: 5–10 • Growing premature infants: 5–15 • Growing term infants: 5–15 • Maximum safe dose:[d] 18

(continued)

Table 2.1 (continued)

Carbohydrate, g/kg/d
- Initial dose: 7
- Transition dose: 8–15
- Growing premature infants: 10–20
- Growing term infants: 8–20
- Maximum safe dose[d]: 25

Protein[e], g/kg/d
- Initial dose: 2–3
- Transition dose: 3.5–4
- Growing premature infants: 3.2–3.8
- Growing term infants: 2.5–3
- Maximum safe dose[d]: 4

Fat[f], g/kg/d
- Initial dose: 0.5–1
- Transition dose: 1–3
- Growing premature infants: 0.5–3
- Growing term infants: 0.5–3
- Maximum safe dose[d]: 4

Sodium, mEq/kg/d
- Initial dose: 0–1
- Transition dose: 2–5
- Growing premature infants: 2–4
- Growing term infants: 2–4
- Maximum safe dose[d]: 20

Potassium, mEq/kg/d
- Initial dose: 0–1
- Transition dose: 0–2
- Growing premature infants: 2–3
- Growing term infants: 2–3
- Maximum safe dose[d]: 9

Chloride[g], mEq/kg/d
- Initial dose: 0–1
- Transition dose: 2–7
- Growing premature infants: 2–7
- Growing term infants: 2–7

(continued)

Table 2.1 (continued)

Acetate

- Initial dose: as needed
- Transition dose: as needed
- Growing premature infants: as needed
- Growing term infants: as needed
- Maximum safe dose [d]: 6 mEq/kg/d

Calcium, mEg/kg/d

- Initial dose:1–3
- Transition dose: 2–3
- Growing premature infants: 3
- Growing term infants: 2
- Maximum safe dose [d]: 4

Phosphorus, mM/kg/d

- Initial dose: 0–0.6
- Transition dose: 1.3–2
- Growing premature infants: 1.3–2
- Growing term infants: 1–1.5
- Maximum safe dose [d]: 2

Magnesium, mEq/kg/d

- Initial dose: 0
- Transition dose: 0.2–0.3
- Growing premature infants: 0.2–0.3
- Growing term infants: 0.25–0.5
- Maximum safe dose [d]: 1

Iron[h], mg/kg/d

- Initial dose: —
- Transition dose: —
- Growing premature infants: (0.2)
- Growing term infants: (0.1)
- Maximum safe dose [d]: 1

[a]Basal energy needs (usually equated with resting energy expenditure) assume a thermoneutral environment. Thermal losses during care may increase energy expenditure by 7 to 8 kcal/kg/d. During periods of acute stress, as in sepsis or major surgery, when C-reactive protein (CRP) levels are elevated, energy expenditure may increase by 8 to 10 kcal/kg/d, although tolerance to carbohydrate and fat may decrease. Basal energy needs may be used in the absence of measured energy expenditure to prevent overfeeding until CRP levels are $\leq$ 2 mg/dL.

(continued)

Table 2.1 (continued)

[b]Total parenteral energy needs listed include basal energy needs plus energy for growth (tissue synthesis and stored energy) and activity. Additional energy is not required for digestion or to replace losses in stool that occur with enteral feeding, but additional energy may be needed during recovery periods after sepsis or surgery or during catch-up growth.
[c]Dextrose is usually the greatest contributor to osmolarity in parenteral nutrient solutions. Peripheral venous access requires limiting dextrose to 12.5% concentration. Solutions with osmolarity > 1,000 mOsm/L, when delivered through peripheral venous access, increase risk of tissue damage. Central venous access allows up to 25% dextrose solutions. Infants with hypoglycemia may require more dextrose initially to maintain euglycemia.
[d]Individual tolerance varies based on many factors. See suggestions in text.
[e]Protein needs may vary with diagnoses: 0.8 to 2 g/kg/d for renal failure; 3 to 4 g/kg/d for necrotizing enterocolitis, major surgery, and sepsis.
[f]Minimum fat dose to meet essential fatty acid requirements varies depending on fat source and total energy needs.
[g]Hyperchloridemic acidosis may occur with high chloride intake; adjust electrolytes by including Na or K as acetate if needed.
[h]Many institutions do not routinely include iron in parenteral admixtures due to incompatibility with other nutrients, contraindication during sepsis, and risks associated with overdose with multiple blood transfusions. See text.
Source: Data are from references 1–7.

FLUIDS

Initiation and Advancement

Initial Phase

Fluid intake should initially be restricted to promote normal postnatal diuresis (approximately 10% to 15% of birth weight) while maintaining electrolyte homeostasis (2,8). Postnatal fluid restriction has been associated with increased rate of weight loss and reduced incidence of NEC and PDA (8,9). A meta-analysis of five studies also found trends toward increased risk of dehydration and reduced risk of bronchopulmonary dysplasia, intracranial hemorrhage, and death in the fluid-restricted groups (8). Infants born at an earlier GA may have higher insensible fluid losses resulting in a greater percentage of weight loss compared with infants born small for gestational age (SGA), who have a more mature body composition (1,3,10,11). Duration of the diuresis phase varies but typically is completed by 96 hours of age in the extremely low birth weight (ELBW) infant (12). Baseline fluid needs by birth weight are listed below.

- Weight < 1 kg: 90 to 120 mL/kg/d (more if medically necessary)
- Weight 1 to 1.5 kg: 70 to 90 mL/kg/d
- Weight > 1.5 kg: 60 to 80 mL/kg/d

Fluid needs may vary widely depending on a number of factors, including clinical condition, environment, and organ maturity (especially skin, lungs, and kidneys). Close monitoring of fluid status is required in order to appropriately determine the patient's actual fluid needs. Fluid needs may be *higher* in (10,13):

- infants born at < 28 weeks' gestation,
- infants with abdominal wall defects,
- infants with high-output renal failure,
- or infants receiving care under a radiant warmer or phototherapy.

Fluid needs may be *lower* or purposefully restricted:

- for early prevention of PDA,
- in infants maintained in a humidified environment,
- in infants with oliguric renal failure,
- or in infants undergoing total body cooling.

Transitional Phase

As renal function improves, skin integrity matures, and postnatal diuresis is completed, fluid intake is gradually liberalized as tolerated to achieve volumes necessary to meet nutrient intake goals. The exact duration of this phase varies, but it typically occurs over the first 1 to 2 weeks of life (2,3). Fluid needs may be *higher* in infants remaining on phototherapy. Fluid needs may be *lower* in infants with oliguria/anuria or with significant lung disease. Fluid restriction is not beneficial for treatment of infants with a symptomatic PDA (14).

Growth Phase

Adequate PN generally requires fluid intakes of 130 to 150 mL/kg/d. A concentrated PN solution (dextrose ≥ 15% and amino acids > 3%) may be required if fluids are restricted below these volumes.

Monitoring of Fluid Status

Fluid status should be monitored by evaluating weight changes, fluid intake, urine output, and serum electrolyte levels (particularly sodium and chloride).

- Normal urine output is 1 to 2 mL/kg/h.
- Markers of overhydration may include weight gain (in excess of that expected for age and nutrient intake), increased urine output (> 3 mL/kg/h), hyponatremia, and edema.
- Markers of dehydration may include weight loss in excess of anticipated postnatal diuresis, decreased urine output (< 1 mL/kg/h), hypernatremia, or sunken fontanelle.

AMINO ACIDS (AA)

AA Solutions

The AA profile in pediatric PN solutions mirrors the serum AA profile of breast milk–fed term infants (15). Pediatric solutions contain a small amount of taurine, which may be an essential AA for preterm infants. These solutions also have a lower pH than adult AA solutions, which improves solubility of calcium and phosphorus (16). Pediatric AA solutions may also reduce risk of parenteral nutrition–associated liver disease (PNALD) when compared with standard solutions (15). They are indicated for use in preterm infants and in older infants at risk for osteopenia or PNALD.

Initiation and Advancement

Early administration of AA intake (within the first 24 hours of life) is safe, promotes positive nitrogen balance, and improves glucose tolerance in preterm infants (17–19).

Initial AA intake at a *minimum* of 1.5 to 2 g/kg/d prevents catabolism; however, initial rates of AA as high as 3.6 g/kg/d have been shown to be safe and prevent negative nitrogen balance (17). Advance AA intake as total energy and fluid intake increases to achieve estimated needs, as shown in Table 2.1.

Monitoring

Routine monitoring of parenteral protein tolerance is not indicated unless doses exceed recommended intake or if the infant has renal dysfunction (elevated serum creatinine). AAs are used for both protein synthesis and as an energy source; therefore, blood urea nitrogen (BUN) is not an effective monitor of parenteral protein tolerance. There is no correlation between the quantity of early parenteral protein intake and BUN levels (20).

DEXTROSE

Initiation and Advancement

Parenteral carbohydrate (CHO) must be initiated carefully, as glucose intolerance and decreased insulin sensitivity are common in the first week of life (21). Although it has been common practice to define a wide range of blood glucose values as acceptable for preterm infants (ie, 50 to 200 mg/dL), blood glucose levels > 150 to 180 mg/dL may be associated with increased mortality and morbidities, including sepsis and retinopathy of prematurity (22–24). Evidence is lacking to support the use and safety of tight glucose control in preterm infants (25).

Recommendations for initial CHO infusion are as follows:

- Preterm infants: 6 to 8 g/kg/d (4 to 6 mg/kg/min)
- Term infants: 8 to 12 g/kg/d (6 to 8 mg/kg/min)

Carbohydrate infusion should be advanced cautiously and as the infant demonstrates tolerance to current glucose infusion rate (GIR). When blood glucose is stable and < 120 mg/dL, consider increasing GIR by 1.5 to 3 g/kg/d (1 to 2 mg/kg/min) until goal energy intake is achieved. If blood glucose is mildly elevated (120 to 150 mg/dL), maintain current GIR. Consider a 1.5 to 3 g/kg/d (1 to 2 mg/kg/min) reduction in GIR whenever blood glucose is moderately elevated (150 to 180 mg/dL). Consider insulin use when blood glucose is markedly elevated (> 180 mg/dL) and CHO intake is restricted to < 6 mg/kg/min as a short-term measure to establish euglycemia (22).

Parenteral CHO concentration may be restricted based on IV location, as dextrose contributes significantly to solution osmolality. Generally, dextrose solutions infused through peripheral lines should not exceed a concentration of 12.5% or an osmolality of 1,000 mOsm/kg. If infused through centrally placed lines, maximum dextrose concentration is typically 25%.

Monitoring

Most institutions will have established glucose monitoring protocols based on gestational age and/or risk factors. General recommendations are as follows:

- Monitor blood glucose at least 4 times daily in the first 24 hours of life in infants at risk for glucose intolerance (See Box 2.1).
- Monitor blood glucose at least 1 to 2 times daily as energy intake is advanced to goal.
- Reduce glucose monitoring to 2 to 3 times per week when blood glucose is stable on goal parenteral intake.

Box 2.1 Common Causes of Hypoglycemia and Hyperglycemia

Causes of Hypoglycemia

- Small for gestational age
- Large for gestational age
- Indomethacin therapy (26)
- Rapid discontinuation of IV dextrose

Causes of Hyperglycemia

- Sepsis
- Extreme prematurity
- Surgery/stress
- Malnutrition
- Renal disease
- Excessive dextrose infusion
- Glucocorticoid therapy
- Thiazide diuretic therapy

INTRAVENOUS FAT EMULSIONS (IVFE)

IVFE provide a source of both energy and essential fatty acids to the neonate (27). The amount of IVFE required to meet essential fatty acid deficiency (EFAD) is dependent on lipid product composition and the infant's metabolic state. In general, an IVFE dose of 0.5 to 1 mg/kg/d should be sufficient to prevent EFAD. Doses ranging from 2 to 4 g/kg/d are typically given to provide an energy source and a balanced substrate solution.

IVFE also help protect peripheral veins from the hypertonicity of PN (28–30). Twenty percent IVFE are cleared more rapidly than 10% IVFE as they contain lower amounts of phospholipid per calorie (1–3). Currently, only soy-oil solutions are approved for use in the United States. Other lipid formulations are approved for use in Europe and are occasionally used in the under research protocols. Fish-oil solutions high in n-3 fatty acids (Omegaven) appear to be a promising alternative product to prevent PNALD (31). Another lipid blend containing soy, medium-chain triglycerides (MCT), olive, and fish oils (SMOFlipid) has been associated with a reduction in risk for retinopathy of prematurity (32). Non-soy-based emulsions may also be associated with a lower risk for sepsis (33). Table 2.2 demonstrates the composition of current lipid products.

Table 2.2 Composition of Current Intravenous Lipid Emulsions

Intralipid

Composition: Soybean oil
20% lipid (200 g lipid/L), 2 kcal/mL, 350 mOsm/L
α-Tocopherol: 87 umol/L
Ratio n-6 to n-3 PUFAs: 7:1
% of fatty acids:

- Linoleic: 53%
- Linolenic: 8%
- ARA: 0.1%
- DHA: 0%
- MCT: 0%

Omegaven[a]

Composition: Fish oil
10% lipid (100 g lipid/L), 1.12 kcal/mL, 273 mOsm/L
α-Tocopherol: 505 umol/L
Ratio n-6 to n-3 PUFAs: 1:8
% of fatty acids:

- Linoleic: 4.4%
- Linolenic: 1.8%
- ARA: 2.1%
- DHA: 12.1%
- MCT: 0%

SMOFlipid

Composition: Soybean oil (30%), coconut oil (30%), olive oil (25%), fish oil (15%)
20% lipid (200 g lipid/L), 2 kcal/mL, 380 mOsm/L
α-Tocopherol: 500 umol/L
Ratio n-6 to n-3 PUFAs: 2.5:1
% of fatty acids:

- Linoleic: 18.6%
- Linolenic: 2.3%
- ARA: 0.5%
- DHA: 2.2%
- MCT: 27.8%

(continued)

Table 2.2 (continued)

ClinOleic
Composition: Olive oil (80%), soybean oil (20%)
20% lipid (200 g lipid/L), 2 kcal/mL, 270 mOsm/L
α-Tocopherol: 75 umol/L
Ratio n-6 to n-3 PUFAs: 9:1
% of fatty acids:

- Linoleic: 18.7%
- Linolenic: 2.3%
- ARA: 0.5%
- DHA: 0%
- MCT: 0%

Abbreviations: ARA, arachidonic acid; DHA, docosahexaenoic acid; MCT, medium-chain triglycerides; PUFA, polyunsaturated fatty acids.
[a] Omegaven is not commercially approved in the United States; it is available only for research protocols or for compassionate use. Prior to implementing this product, approval must be obtained from the US Food and Drug Administration (FDA) (www.fda.gov).
Source: Data are from references 27 and 33.

Administration of IVFE in a total nutrient admixture (TNA) is not indicated for neonatal PN because lipid stability is decreased by the hypertonic, acidic, and high mineral (particularly calcium) content of these solutions (34,35). Additionally, the presence of precipitates or other particulates may be masked by the opacity of TNAs. Studies using multichamber bags instead of TNAs have been completed in Europe and are promising (36).

Initiation and Advancement

IVFE may be initiated within the first 24 to 48 hours of life (1,3,33). Advance lipids as needed to meet energy goals (See Table 2.1). IVFE infused over 20 to 24 hours promote optimal clearance.

Special Conditions and Administration of IVFE

- Hyperbilirubinemia: Restriction of IVFE is not indicated in infants with neonatal jaundice because doses up to 3.25 g/kg/d do not displace bilirubin from albumin (37).
- Pulmonary Hypertension: Delayed initiation and cautious advancement may be indicated because IVFE can increase pulmonary vascular resistance (38).
- Sepsis: Restriction of IVFE to 1 g/kg/d while blood culture is positive has been associated with a faster return to a negative blood culture but can also be associated with a slower rate of weight gain (39).
- PNALD: Restriction of IVFE is controversial; see Chronic Complications, later in this chapter.

Monitoring

Monitor triglyceride levels in infants receiving > 2 g/kg/d IVFE. If serum triglyceride level exceeds 250 mg/dL, a reduction in lipid intake by 0.5 to 1 g/kg/d or an increase in levocarnitine dose to improve fatty acid oxidation may be warranted. Infants who are dependent on PN and restricted to ≤ 1 g/kg IVFE and who demonstrate poor growth may benefit from screening of fatty acid levels or a triene:tetraene ratio to rule out EFAD.

ELECTROLYTES

Dose recommendations are given in Table 2.1. Monitoring recommendations are given in Table 2.3 (3).

Table 2.3 Recommended Frequency of Electrolyte and Acid/Base (Blood Gas) Monitoring

Conditions	Frequency of Monitoring
Postnatal diuresis (age ~3–8 d) and/or advancement to goal PN	Daily
At goal PN with stable, normal electrolytes and acid/base status	1–2 times per week
PN > 3 weeks with normal electrolytes and acid/base status	Every 1–2 weeks

Abbreviation: PN, parenteral nutrition.
Source: Data are from reference 3.

Sodium (40)

Sodium may be present in PN solutions as chloride, acetate, and/or phosphate. Sodium should be limited to 0 to 1 mEq/kg/d until postnatal diuresis has been achieved. Restriction of sodium intake to < 0 to 1 mEq/kg/d during the first few days of life has been associated with a reduced incidence of bronchopulmonary dysplasia. Advance sodium intake to between 2 and 3 mEq/kg when infant begins to regain birth weight.

Extremely premature infants may require higher sodium intakes due to limited renal tubular sodium reabsorption. If hydration status is stable, adjust sodium intake by 1 to 2 mEq/kg/d as needed to maintain normal serum sodium values. Late-onset hyponatremia may require 5 to 7 mEq/kg/d.

Potassium

Potassium may be present in PN solutions as chloride, acetate, or less often as phosphate. Provide potassium-free PN until urine output is well established (> 1 mL/kg/h) and serum potassium is within normal limits. Advance potassium intake to 2 to 3 mEq/kg/d and adjust as needed based on changes in renal function or changes in serum values, particularly with use of diuretic medications.

Because early initiation of amino acids leads to positive nitrogen balance, infants now require supplemental potassium in the first days of life to prevent hypokalemia. This situation is particularly true in infants born with intrauterine growth restriction (IUGR) who are at risk for refeeding syndrome (41). Early and frequent monitoring of potassium may be indicated in this population.

Nonoliguric hyperkalemia is also a potential early complication of extremely premature infants. Incidence of this condition has declined with earlier administration of AAs and better management of fluids. Although the cause of nonoliguric hyperkalemia is unknown, factors that may exacerbate this condition include extreme prematurity, bruising, blood group incompatibility, catabolism, metabolic acidosis, and excessive potassium intake.

Chloride and Acetate

Chloride and additional acetate intake should be restricted until the neonate is ready for the inclusion of sodium and potassium additives to PN. Limit chloride to 2 to 3 mEq/kg/d to prevent hyperchloremic acidosis. If sodium requirement exceeds 5 mEq/kg/d, higher intakes of chloride may be given, up to 7 mEq/kg/d.

The presence of acetate in PN reduces the incidence of hyperchloremic metabolic acidosis (42). Pediatric AA solutions contain approximately 1 mEq acetate per g of protein equivalent. Sodium and potassium may also be given as acetate, but total acetate intake (including the acetate present in the AA base solution) should generally not exceed 6 mEq/kg/d.

CALCIUM AND PHOSPHORUS

Dose Recommendations

Estimated requirements for calcium and phosphorus are given in Table 2.1. Calcium is typically provided as calcium gluconate, while phosphorus may be added as either sodium phosphate or potassium phosphate. Phosphate additives contain differing amounts of phosphorus per mEq of cation; sodium phosphate contains 1.33 mEq sodium, while potassium phosphate contains 1.5 mEq potassium for each mMol of phosphorus.

The ideal calcium-to-phosphorus ratio to promote optimal mineral retention and tolerance is as follows:

- 1.3 to 1.7 mg calcium: 1 mg phosphorus, or
- 1 to 1.3 mMol calcium: 1 mMol phosphorus, or
- 2.2 to 2.6 mEq calcium: 1 mMol phosphorus (units frequently used in PN compounding)

Mineral wasting or alterations in mineral homeostasis may be caused by alternate-day calcium and phosphorus infusions or with ratios *less* than:

- 1 mg calcium:1 mg phosphorus, or
- 0.8 mMol calcium:1 mMol phosphorus, or
- 1.6 mEq calcium:1 mMol phosphorus

Calcium needs may be higher in infants with increased urinary calcium loss due to medications such as diuretics (especially furosemide), theophylline, and steroids (43). Early parenteral needs for phosphorus are positively associated with the level of parenteral AA intake (44). Phosphorus needs may also be increased in infants with IUGR and those born to mothers with preeclampsia, as these infants demonstrate signs of refeeding syndrome in the setting of rapid growth (41). Early and frequent monitoring of phosphorus may be indicated in this population.

Barriers to Mineral Provision

Calcium and phosphorus intake in neonatal PN is limited due to conditions of mineral solubility. Factors that *improve* calcium and phosphorus solubility include the following:

- Higher acidity of neonatal AA solutions (compared with standard adult AA solutions)
- Presence of cysteine hydrochloride additive
- Higher concentrations of AAs and dextrose
- Lipids administered separately

Factors that *reduce* calcium and phosphorus solubility include the following:

- Higher concentrations of calcium and phosphorus
- Lower concentrations of protein or dextrose
- Lack of cysteine hydrochloride additive
- Higher environmental temperatures
- Lipids administered in a TNA

Check with pharmacy to determine maximal allowable mineral concentrations for specific PN solutions.

Monitoring

As PN advances, ionized calcium and phosphorus should be monitored 1 to 2 times weekly to evaluate adequacy of calcium:phosphorus ratio in SGA infants and premature infants born < 32 weeks' gestation. Alkaline phosphatase should also be monitored in infants on PN > 2 weeks to evaluate for development of osteopenia (see Chapter 15, Osteopenia of Prematurity). Hepatic sources of alkaline phosphatase may also be elevated when cholestasis is present, which may confound interpretation of serum levels of this enzyme. In general, an elevated alkaline phosphatase in the presence of PNALD is reflective of mineral deficiency, not liver disease (45). Levels, however, may be fractionated or assessed for isoenzymes to determine whether the enzyme source is likely to be bone or hepatic.

MAGNESIUM

Estimated requirements for magnesium are listed in Table 2.1. Magnesium may be omitted from initial and/or transitional PN if the mother received significant amounts of antenatal magnesium sulfate.

VITAMINS

Dose Recommendations

Goals for vitamin intake are shown in Table 2.4.

Table 2.4 Estimated Daily Parenteral Vitamin Requirements and Dose Recommendations for Preterm Infants

Vitamin	Recommended Amount	Delivered Amount Using Dose Recommendations Based on Infant Weight[b]
Vitamin A, IU/kg/d	700–1500	• 0.5–1 kg: 700–1400 • 1–2.5 kg: 600–1500 • ≤ 2.5 kg: 920 • > 2.5 kg: 2300
Vitamin D, IU/kg/d	40–160	• 0.5–1 kg: 120–240 • 1–2.5 kg: 100–260 • ≤ 2.5 kg: 160 • > 2.5 kg: 400
Vitamin E, IU/kg/d	2.8–3.5	• 0.5–1 kg: 2.1–4.2 • 1–2.5 kg: 1.8–4.5 • ≤ 2.5 kg: 2.8 • > 2.5 kg: 7

(continued)

Table 2.4 Estimated Daily Parenteral Vitamin Requirements and Dose Recommendations for Preterm Infants (continued)

Vitamin K, mcg/kg/d	10–100	• 0.5–1 kg: 60–120 • 1–2.5 kg: 50–130 • ≤ 2.5 kg: 80 • > 2.5 kg: 200
Thiamin, mcg/kg/d	200–350	• 0.5–1 kg: 360–720 • 1–2.5 kg: 312–780 • ≤ 2.5 kg: 480 • > 2.5 kg: 1200
Riboflavin, mcg/kg/d	150–200	• 0.5–1 kg: 420–840 • 1–2.5 kg: 364–910 • ≤ 2.5 kg: 560 • > 2.5 kg: 1400
Niacin, mg/kg/d	4–6.8	• 0.5–1 kg: 5–10 • 1–2.5 kg: 4.4–11 • ≤ 2.5 kg: 6.8 • > 2.5 kg: 17
Vitamin B-6, mcg/kg/d	150–200	• 0.5–1 kg: 300–600 • 1–2.5 kg: 260–650 • ≤ 2.5 kg: 400 • > 2.5 kg: 1,000
Folate, mcg/kg/d	56	• 0.5–1 kg: 42–84 • 1–2.5 kg: 36–90 • ≤ 2.5 kg: 56 • > 2.5 kg: 140
Vitamin B-12, mcg/kg/d	0.3	• 0.5–1 kg: 0.3–0.6 • 1–2.5 kg: 0.3–0.6 • ≤ 2.5 kg: 0.4 • > 2.5 kg: 1
d-Panthenol, mg/kg/d	1–2	• 0.5–1 kg: 1.5–3 • 1–2.5 kg: 1.3–3.3 • ≤ 2.5 kg: 2 • > 2.5 kg: 5

(continued)

Table 2.4 (continued)

Biotin, mcg/kg/d	5–8	• 0.5–1 kg: 6–12 • 1–2.5 kg: 5–13 • ≤ 2.5 kg: 8 • > 2.5 kg: 20
Vitamin C, mg/kg/d	15–25	• 0.5–1 kg: 24–48 • 1–2.5 kg: 21–52 • ≤ 2.5 kg: 32 • > 2.5 kg: 80

[a]Amounts listed are for both pediatric multivitamin preparations: Pediatric MVI Injection or Unit Vial, Astra USA, Inc, Westboro, MA 01581-4500 and INFUVIT Pediatric, Sabex Inc, Boucherville, QC, Canada J4B 7K8.

[b] Dose recommendations by infant weight:

- 0.5–1 kg: 1.5 mL/d (30% dose/d)
- 1–2.5 kg: 3.25 mL/d (65% dose/d)
- ≤ 2.5 kg: 2 mL/kg/d (40% dose/kg/d)
- > 2.5 kg: 5 mL/d (100% dose/d)

Doses based on 1 full dose = 5 mL. Maximum dose not to exceed 1 full 5 mL dose per day.

Source: Data are from references 1–3, 7, 46, and 49.

Pediatric multivitamin solutions provide more appropriate levels of vitamins than adult multivitamin preparations, but they are relatively high in water-soluble vitamins and low in vitamin A. Water-soluble vitamins are photosensitive and may degrade and oxidize upon exposure to light (47–49). Although the clinical significance of this effect is still being evaluated, protection of PN bags and tubing from light exposure seems to minimize this process.

Monitoring

Routine monitoring of vitamin levels is not usually recommended. As the infant is weaned from PN and enteral feeds provide a greater proportion of total vitamin intake, monitoring of fat-soluble vitamin levels (especially vitamin D), vitamin B-12, and/or prothrombin times may be indicated depending on the patient's clinical condition.

TRACE ELEMENTS

Dose Recommendations

Trace element requirements are less thoroughly researched for neonates than for other age groups. Specific parenteral dose recommendations, however, are available for zinc, copper, manganese, chromium, selenium, and iron. Recommendations are based on GA, postnatal age, and clinical condition. See Table 2.5.

Table 2.5 Estimated Parenteral Trace Element Requirements for Preterm Infants

Dosing Category	Estimated Requirements, mcg/kg/d
Initial stabilization period[a]	Zinc: 150 Copper: 0–10 Manganese: 0–1 Chromium: 0–0.1 Selenium: 0–1.3
Growing preterm infant, birth to term	Zinc: 400 Copper: 20 Manganese: 1.0 Chromium: 0.1 Selenium: 1.5–2[b]
Growing term infant, birth to 3 mo	Zinc: 250 Copper: 20 Manganese: 1.0 Chromium: 0.1 Selenium: 2[b]
Cholestasis, direct bilirubin > 2 mg/dL	Zinc: • Preterm: 400 • Term: 250 • 3 mo: 100 Copper: 20 Manganese: 0 Chromium: 0.1 Selenium: 2[b]

(continued)

Table 2.5 Estimated Parenteral Trace Element Requirements for Preterm Infants (continued)

Renal insufficiency, creatinine > 1 mg/dL (undialyzed)	Zinc: • Preterm: 400 • Term: 250 • High-output failure: 600 Copper: 20 Manganese: 1.0 Chromium: 0 Selenium: 0
Specific Products	**Dose Provides (in mcg/kg/d)**
Multitrace Neonatal[c] dose: 0.2 mL/kg/d	Zinc: 300 Copper: 20 Manganese: 5 Chromium: 0.17 Selenium: 0
Multitrace Pediatric[c] dose: 0.2 mL/kg/d	Zinc: 200 Copper: 20 Manganese: 5 Chromium: 0.2 Selenium: 0
Multitrace Pediatric[c] dose: 0.1 mL/kg/d	Zinc: 100 Copper: 10 Manganese: 2.5 Chromium: 0.1 Selenium: 0

[a]Stabilization period varies by reference: Day 0–7, Day 0–10, or Day 0–14.
[b]For infants older than 28 days.
[c]Nutrient content listed is per manufacturer's label (American Regent, Inc, Shirley, NY 11967). Always check current product information before administering.
Source: Data are from references 1–3, 7, 46, and 49.

None of the available neonatal or pediatric trace element packages meet the needs of every age or clinical condition; manganese content within trace element packages may be 5 times the recommended dose when other elements are administered at recommended doses.

Recommendations for changes in trace element products and dosing were published in 2012 (49). Trace elements are available separately and may be dosed individually instead of within a package (see Table 2.5).

Individual Trace Element Considerations (1,2,7,50)

Zinc

Zinc deficiency has been described in neonates of various birth weights and gestational ages. Low serum levels of zinc (< 74 mcg/dL) are diagnostic for deficiency, although zinc levels may be falsely normal or elevated during tissue catabolism or times of increased bone tissue turnover. Symptoms of zinc deficiency may include:

- anorexia
- failure to thrive
- weight loss
- decreased linear growth
- dermatitis (particularly around mucous membranes)
- diarrhea
- alopecia
- increased susceptibility to infection
- impaired wound healing
- hypoproteinemia with generalized edema
- reduced alkaline phosphatase enzyme level

Zinc requirements may be higher in certain clinical conditions; increased loss due to high-output renal failure may require intakes of 600 mcg/kg/d. Because zinc is primarily absorbed in the proximal small bowel, and enterohepatic recirculation of zinc is considerable in the distal small bowel, patients with short bowel syndrome or with increased stool/ostomy loss may require up to 800 mcg/kg/d.

Copper

It has previously been recommended to reduce or remove copper from parenteral solutions if PNALD is present; however, copper deficiency has been observed with this practice (51,52). Although copper is excreted in bile, hepatic tissue levels of copper decrease as liver disease progresses, indicating a possible protective role. Current recommendations are to reduce or remove copper only if evidence of toxicity is present.

Manganese

Manganese is excreted primarily in bile, but serum manganese is elevated in patients with cholestatic jaundice and is directly correlated to the severity of cholestasis. Manganese contamination of PN additives may provide sufficient daily intake without additional supplementation. Manganese should be removed from PN when direct bilirubin is > 2 mg/dL, especially if enteral intake is minimal and slow advancement of enteral intake is anticipated. Excessive intake of parenteral manganese may induce PNALD and neurotoxicity (53,54).

Selenium and Chromium

Selenium and chromium requirements may be decreased in patients with chronic (undialyzed) renal failure. The selenium dose may be reduced to 1 mcg/kg/d or omitted, and chromium may be omitted (see Table 2.5) (46).

Iodine

A meta-analysis of iodine supplementation in preterm infants found insufficient evidence to recommend the practice at this time (55). Because cutaneous and IV solution contaminant iodine are no longer considered significant sources, some neonatologists recommend the addition of iodine to PN (56). A reasonable dose is 10 mcg/kg/d (56).

Monitoring

Routine monitoring of trace element status is not indicated. For infants with PNALD, monitoring every 1 to 3 months for serum copper, ceruloplasmin, and whole blood manganese may help identify toxicity. Once these trace elements have been removed or reduced, monitoring is indicated to evaluate for adequacy of intake. Infants with increased GI losses or unexplained growth failure may warrant measurement of serum zinc.

RECOMMENDATIONS FOR OTHER NUTRIENTS

Cysteine

Cysteine is often added to PN solutions, although its role as an essential AA for preterm infants remains controversial. The addition of cysteine to PN does not improve growth, although nitrogen retention is increased (57). Cysteine reduces the pH of the PN solution, thus enhancing the solubility of calcium and phosphorus (9). The recommended dose for cysteine hydrochloride is 40 mg per g of AA (2,3). This dose, however, may promote metabolic acidosis; acid/base status should be closely monitored and acetate content of cysteine-containing PN solutions should be increased as needed to promote homeostasis (58).

Carnitine

Serum carnitine levels decrease rapidly in preterm infants during the first 2 weeks of PN (59). A clinical benefit of routine carnitine supplementation of neonatal PN has not been identified (60). Carnitine supplementation may be beneficial, however, for infants receiving nutrition solely via PN for an extended period of time. The estimated requirement of carnitine is between 2 and 10 mg/kg/d (1–3).

Iron

Iron is not recommended as a routine additive to neonatal PN due to concerns of iron toxicity and oxidative injury (See Table 2.1). Oral supplementation of iron is a safer alternative for infants receiving a significant amount of enteral nutrition. The addition of 0.1 to 0.2 mg/kg/d of parenteral iron may be indicated for infants in whom iron deficiency develops, or for those dependent solely on PN for longer than 2 months, especially if measures to avoid blood transfusions are taken (eg, a Jehovah's Witness family) (2,3).

OTHER ADDITIVES

Heparin

Heparin has been shown to reduce risk of catheter thrombosis in arterial lines (61). Studies have not shown conclusive benefits to the addition of heparin to peripheral intravenous catheters or peripherally inserted central catheters (PICCs) (62,63). Higher doses of heparin (83.5 units/kg vs 59.4 units/kg) have been associated with an increased risk of intraventricular hemorrhage (64).

Insulin

Insulin is not recommended as a routine additive to PN, although hyperglycemia may be associated with increased morbidity (65,66). Insulin may be indicated for infants who demonstrate a significant elevation in serum glucose with intakes < 50 to 60 kcal/kg/d or GIR of < 6 mg/kg/min (2,3,67,68).

In neonates, insulin should be infused separately from the PN solution, as insulin dose may change frequently with medical status and advancing age. The use of insulin solely to increase nutrient intake to levels that exceed normal requirements warrants further investigation.

ADDITIONAL PN CONSIDERATIONS

Starter PN

Starter PN solution (also known as "vanilla" PN) is standardized and premixed for initial parenteral feeding (69). It is initiated as soon as IV access is established (within the first hours of life), and is continued until custom PN is ordered. Starter PN solution may be infused at 50 to 80 mL/kg/d and should provide maintenance CHO intake and 1.5 to 3 g/kg/d AA. To increase flexibility for use and to extend the shelf life of this product, starter PN typically does not include lipids, electrolyte additives, trace elements, or vitamins; some institutions include between 5 and 20 mEq of calcium gluconate per liter.

PN During Periods of Fluid, Glucose, and Electrolyte Imbalance

Infants born at < 26 weeks' gestation often show alterations in fluid, glucose, and electrolyte tolerance in the first few days of life. To ensure prescribed doses of AA and minerals are infused, it may be beneficial to use a more concentrated PN solution at between 50 and 80 mL/kg/d; additional IV fluids may be rapidly adjusted as glucose, fluid, and electrolyte status changes. As conditions stabilize, PN volume can be advanced to supply all IV fluid needs.

PN During Initiation and Progression of Enteral Feedings

Nutrient intakes and rate of growth have been shown to decline during the transition from full parenteral to full enteral feedings (70). Relative nutrient densities of enteral and parenteral feeds should be taken into consideration during this transition. Ideally, the nutrient composition of PN should be adjusted to complement the nutrient composition of enteral feeds in order to meet overall intake goals.

CHRONIC COMPLICATIONS (71)

PNALD (72)

Risk Factors

Risk factors for PNALD, which is also known as parenteral nutrition-associated cholestasis (PNAC) or cholestasis (direct bilirubin > 2 mg/dL), include:

- lack of enteral feeds > 21 days (73)
- sepsis (particularly gram-negative bacteria) (74)
- SGA (51,75)
- overfeeding of parenteral nutrients, particularly dextrose and lipid (76)
- IVFE rich in phytosterols (soy oil) (77)

Prevention/Treatment

Restriction of IVFE to 1 g/kg/d is common practice in infants with cholestasis (direct bilirubin >2 mg/dL); however, the efficacy of this practice is controversial and requires additional monitoring for EFAD (78–82).

- Initiate trophic enteral feeds as soon as clinically appropriate.
- Provide adequate, but not excessive amounts of macronutrients (protein intake to meet needs for age and

clinical condition, 60% to 70% of nonprotein calories as CHO, and 30% to 40% as fat).

- Consider cyclic administration of PN.
- Consider use of ursodeoxycholic acid when enteral feeds are tolerated (83).
- Use pediatric AA preparations that contain taurine (84).
- Consider a fish oil–based IVFE if available (85).

Metabolic Bone Disease (Osteopenia of Prematurity)

Metabolic bone disease, also referred to as osteopenia of prematurity, is identified by the appearance of reduced bone mineralization on x-ray, or an alkaline phosphatase > 900 IU/L and a serum phosphorus < 5.6 mg/dL (86,87).

Risk Factors

Risk factors for metabolic disease include the following:

- Extended period of PN
- Extended use of unfortified breast milk or term infant formula
- Chronic use of diuretics or steroids
- Chronic use of phenobarbital (due to interaction with vitamin D)
- Vitamin D deficiency

Treatment

- Use pediatric AA solutions and additional cysteine hydrochloride.
- Collaborate with pharmacy to maximize mineral content of PN.
- Optimize mineral content of enteral feeds (See Chapters 3 and 4).
- Consider enteral vitamin D supplementation.

ADMINISTRATION ISSUES

Aluminum Toxicity

Aluminum toxicity may occur from aluminum contamination of PN additives. Infants at highest risk are those with increased calcium and phosphorus needs and those on extended courses of TPN. Calcium and phosphorus are the greatcst sources of aluminum, but multivitamin and trace element additives also contain appreciable amounts. Calcium gluconate contains high levels of aluminum contaminants, but alternative calcium sources (calcium chloride, calcium glubionate) have limited solubility when infused with phosphorus. Other sources of aluminum include heparin, albumin, and some IV medications (88). Aluminum toxicity may be associated with metabolic bone disease, hypochromic microcytic anemia, and neurotoxicity (86,88). The US Food and Drug Administration (FDA) has established guidelines for aluminum content of PN components and recommends maintaining aluminum intake between < 4 and 5 mcg/kg/d (89).

Prevention

- Encourage enteral intake to reduce need for PN.
- Monitor parenteral additives, selecting products that contain the lowest amount of aluminum contaminants.
- Use sodium phosphate instead of potassium phosphate.
- Select additives packaged in plastic instead of glass.
- Encourage rapid turnover of additives packaged in glass. Aluminum is a contaminant in glass and leaches into the additive over time.

Access

PN may be administered through a variety of IV sites and catheters (See Box 2.2) (30,90,91). Routine x-ray monitors of central catheter tip location is indicated because lines may migrate over time, especially as the infant grows or demonstrates changes in hydration.

Box 2.2 Access for Parenteral Nutrition

Peripheral Access[a]

- Maintain osmolality of solution 300–1000 mOsm/kg water
- Limit dextrose concentration to ≤ 12.5%
- Co-infuse lipids to help protect line integrity (30)

Central Access[b]

Peripherally inserted central venous catheter (PICC):

- Insertion via peripheral vein, threaded into the central circulation
- Monitor catheter tip location weekly as catheter may kink, occlude, or migrate over time
- Adjust osmolality and dextrose concentration of PN if tip is no longer centrally located
- Consider addition of heparin to minimize risk of developing thrombus

Central venous catheters (CVC):

- Ideal for infants who are likely to require PN for extended periods of time
- CVCs allow direct access to central circulation, but pose a high risk of septicemia
- Maximal dextrose concentration recommendations vary, but typically do not exceed 25%

Umbilical artery catheter (UAC) and umbilical venous catheter (UVC):

- UACs are not commonly used for PN delivery, but are usually saved for lab and blood pressure monitoring (90)
- UVCs are commonly used for PN delivery; however, use for > 7 days may increase risk for central line-associated blood stream infection (CLABSI) (91)
- Maximal dextrose concentration may vary depending on tip position relative to renal and hepatic vessels

[a]For short-term use.

[b]For extended use and safe administration of solutions with greater osmolality and dextrose concentration.

Source: Data are from references 30, 90, and 91.

Osmolality

In animal models, thrombophlebitis is associated with low pH and increased osmolality of parenteral solutions—both are common characteristics of neonatal PN (92). Pediatric patients receiving peripherally infused PN with an osmolality of >1,000 mOsm/kg have an increased risk for infiltration and/or a combined end point of phlebitis and infiltration (93). For this reason, it seems prudent to limit parenteral osmolality to < 1,000 mOsm/kg and to co-infuse IVFE to further dilute osmolality in infants with peripheral access (30).

Line Filters

Line filters have been suggested to minimize the risk of both bacterial contamination and infusion of IV particulates. A meta-analysis found no significant effect of the use of in-line filters on morbidity or mortality of neonates; however, the studies were few and limited in size (94). A prospective, randomized trial of pediatric intensive care patients found that systemic inflammatory response syndrome (SIRS) and length of intensive care unit stay were reduced in patients receiving in-line filtration (95).

Cyclic Administration

In cyclic administration, PN is infused for < 24 hours each day with a 4- to 8-hour interruption in nutrient delivery. Providing a diurnal cycle of PN may help decrease circulating levels of insulin and may protect hepatocytes from excessive glycogen and lipid deposition. In addition, cyclic PN offers opportunities for increased activity levels by allowing physical freedom from IV lines and infusion pumps. This method of nutrition support is most appropriate for infants at or near their term-adjusted age with anticipated long-term need for PN and existing PNALD.

Surgical infants (with anticipated need for extended PN course) may also benefit from initiation of cyclic PN *prior* to development of PNALD (96).

There are no established guidelines for the maximum GIR acceptable in cyclic PN. Carbohydrate infusion must be individualized based on an infant's nutrient requirements, degree of enteral intake, and history of glucose tolerance on continuous PN. Transition to a cyclic regimen requires close monitoring of tolerance. To prevent hypoglycemia when interrupting PN, the infusion is tapered for a period of time, usually at half the full rate, for 30 to 60 minutes. Infusion is restarted gradually, usually at half the full rate, for 30 to 60 minutes, to prevent hyperglycemia when PN resumes. Most current home infusion pumps have a built-in taper feature that will automatically adjust infusion rate. Young infants may demonstrate wider fluctuations in blood glucose levels when they are on cyclic PN. For these infants, the initial "off PN" interval should be brief (2 hours) and increased slowly (eg, by 1 to 2 hours) as tolerance is demonstrated. If clinically appropriate, it may also be beneficial to provide enteral nutrition during the "off PN" interval.

Product Shortages

Shortages of PN additives have occurred frequently over the last 5 years. These shortages may increase the risk for impaired growth and nutrient deficiencies in neonates who have increased nutrient needs and dependence on PN (97). The American Society for Parenteral and Enteral Nutrition (A.S.P.E.N.) has published recommendations for institutions dealing with PN shortages, and it updates recommendations on its website (www.nutritioncare.org) as circumstances change (98). The following are general suggestions for PN for neonates during periods of product shortages:

- Use neonatal and pediatric products for neonates and pediatric patients only.
- Use enteral supplements whenever possible.
- Prioritize patients at highest risk for provision of the product under shortage.
- Avoid use of parenteral products as enteral supplements.
- Prepare PN in a centralized location to limit product waste.
- Consider use of individual nutrient additives instead of multinutrient packages when applicable.
- Consider alternative sources for parenteral products when approved by FDA. (Review differences in product composition before implementation.)
- Monitor for nutrient deficiencies during periods of product shortage.

SUMMARY

The information in this chapter is not meant to be an exhaustive exposition of PN in the neonate, but rather a practical guide or reference for providing fluids and nutrients during the initial days after birth and throughout the neonatal period. Additional information is available in the references listed for this chapter.

REFERENCES

1. Groh-Wargo S, Thompson M, Cox JH. *Nutritional Care for High-Risk Newborns.* 3rd ed. Chicago, IL: Precept Press; 2000.
2. Koletzko B, Poindexter B, Uauy R, eds. In Koletzko B, Poindexter B, Uauy R, eds. *Nutritional Care of Preterm Infants: Scientific Basis and Practical Guidelines*. Basel, Switzerland: Karger; 2014. *World Review of Nutrition and Dietetics*. vol 110.

3. Tsang RC, Uauy R, Koletzko B, Zlotkin SH, eds. *Nutrition of the Preterm Infant Scientific Basis and Practical Guidelines*. 2nd ed. Cincinnati, OH: Digital Education Publishing; 2005.
4. Pierro A. Metabolism and nutritional support in the surgical neonate. *J Pediatr Surg*. 2002;37:811–822.
5. Chwals WJ. Energy expenditure in critically ill neonates. *Pediatr Crit Care Med*. 2008;9:121–122.
6. Ziegler EE. Meeting the nutritional needs of the low-birth-weight-infant. *Ann Nutr Metab*. 2011;58(Suppl 1):8–18.
7. Nutritional needs of the preterm infant. In: Kleinman RE, Greer FR, eds. *Pediatric Nutrition*. 7th ed. Elk Grove Village, IL: American Academy of Pediatrics; 2014:83–121.
8. Oh W, Poindexter BB, Perritt R, Lemons JA, Bauer CR, Ehrenkranz RA, Stoll BJ, Poole K, Wright LL; Neonatal Research Network. Association between fluid intake and weight loss during the first ten days of life and risk of bronchopulmonary dysplasia in extremely low birth weight infants. *J Pediatr*. 2005;147:786–790.
9. Bell EF, Acarregui MJ. Restricted versus liberal water intake for preventing morbidity and mortality in preterm infants. *Cochrane Database Syst Rev*. 2008;(1):CD000503.
10. Grünhagen DJ, de Boer MG, de Beaufort AJ, Walther FJ. Transepidermal water loss during halogen spotlight phototherapy in preterm infants. *Pediatr Res*. 2002;51:402–405.
11. Wadhawan R, Oh W, Perritt R, Laptook AR, Poole K, Wright LL, Fanaroff AA, Duara S, Stoll BJ, Goldberg R. Association between early postnatal weight loss and death or BPD in small and appropriate for gestational age extremely low-birth-weight infants. *J Perinatol*. 2007;27:359–364.
12. Lorenz JM, Kleinman LI, Ahmed G, Markarian K. Phases of fluid and electrolyte homeostasis in the extremely low birth weight infant. *Pediatrics*. 1995;96(3 Pt 1):484–489.
13. Maayan-Metzger A, Yosipovitch G, Hada E, Sirota L. Effect of radiant warmer on transepidermal water loss (TEWL) and skin hydration in preterm infants. *J Perinatol*. 2004;24(6):372–375.
14. De Buyst J, Rakza T, Pennaforte T, Johansson AB, Storme L. Hemodynamic effects of fluid restriction in preterm infants with significant patent ductus arteriosus. *J Pediatr*. 2012;161:404–408.
15. Heird WC, Dell RB, Helms RA, Greene HL, Ament ME, Karna P, Storm MC. Amino acid mixture designed to maintain normal

plasma amino acid patterns in infants and children requiring parenteral nutrition. *Pediatrics.* 1987;80:401–408.

16. Lenz GT, Mikrut BA. Calcium and phosphate solubility in neonatal parenteral nutrient solutions containing Aminosyn-PF or TrophAmine. *Am J Hosp Pharm.* 1988;45(11):2367–2371.
17. Vlaardingerbroek H, Roelants JA, Rook D, Dorst K, Schierbeek H, Vermes A, Vermeulen MJ, van Goudoever JB, van den Akker CH. Adaptive regulation of amino acid metabolism on early parenteral lipid and high-dose amino acid administration in VLBW infants – A randomized controlled trial. *Clin Nutr.* 2014;33:982–990.
18. Ehrenkranz RA. Early, aggressive nutritional management for very low birth weight infants: what is the evidence? *Semin Perinatol.* 2007;31:48–55.
19. Burattini I, Bellagamba MP, Spagnoli C, D'Ascenzo R, Mazzoni N, Peretti A, Cogo PE, Carnielli VP; Marche Neonatal Network. Targeting 2.5 versus 4 g/kg/d of amino acids for extremely low birth weight infants: a randomized clinical trial. *J Pediatr.* 2013;163:1278–1282.
20. Ridout E, Melara D, Rottinghaus S, Thureen PJ. Blood urea nitrogen concentration as a marker of amino-acid intolerance in neonates with birthweight less than 1250 g. *J Perinatol.* 2005;25:130–133.
21. Decaro M, Vain N. Hyperglycaemia in preterm neonates: what to know, what to do. *Early Hum Dev.* 2011;87 Suppl 1:S19–S22.
22. Kao LS, Morris BH, Lally KP, Stewart CD, Huseby V, Kennedy KA. Hyperglycemia and morbidity and mortality in extremely low birth weight infants. *J Perinatol.* 2006;26:730–736.
23. Mohsen L, Abou-Alam M, El-Dib, Labib M, Elsada M, Aly H. A prospective study on hyperglycemia and retinopathy of prematurity. *J Perinatol.* 2014;34(6):453–457.
24. Heimann K, Peschgens T, Kwiecien R, Stanzel S, Hoernchen H, and Merz U. Are recurrent hyperglycemic episodes and median blood glucose level a prognostic factor for increased morbidity and mortality in premature infants ≤1500 g? *J Perinat Med.* 2007;35:245–248.
25. Sinclair JC, Bottino M, Cowett RM. Interventions for prevention of neonatal hyperglycemia in very low birth weight infants. *Cochrane Database Syst Rev.* 2011;(10):CD007615. doi: 10.1002/14651858.CD007615.pub3.
26. Hosono S, Ohno T, Kimoto H, Nagoshi R, Shimizu M, Nozawa M. Reduction in blood glucose values following

indomethacin therapy for patent ductus arteriosus. *Pediatr Int.* 1999;41:525–528.

27. Putet G. Lipid metabolism of the micropremie. *Clin Perinatol.* 2000;27(1):57–69.
28. Koo WWK, McLaughlin K, Saba M. Neonatal intensive care. In: Merritt RJ, ed. *The A.S.P.E.N. Nutrition Support Practice Manual.* 2nd ed. Silver Spring, MD: American Society for Parenteral and Enteral Nutrition; 2005:301–314.
29. Adamkin DH. Use of intravenous lipids in very low-birth weight infants. *Neoreviews.* 2007;12:e543–e545.
30. Pineault M, Chessex P, Piedboeuf B, Bisaillon S. Beneficial effect of coinfusing a lipid emulsion on venous patency. *JPEN J Parenter Enteral Nutr.* 1989;13:637–640.
31. Nandivada P, Carlson SJ, Cowan E, Chang MI, Gura KM, Puder M. Role of parenteral lipid emulsions in the preterm infant. *Early Hum Dev.* 2013;89(Suppl 2):S45–S49.
32. Beken S, Dilli D, Fettah ND, Kabatas EU, Zenciroglu A, Okumus N. The influence of fish-oil lipid emulsions on retinopathy of prematurity in very low birth weight infants: a randomized controlled trial. *Early Hum Dev*. 2014;90:27–31.
33. Vlaardingerbroek H, Veldhorst MAB, Spronk S, van den Akker C, van Goudoever JB. Parenteral lipid administration to very-low-birth-weight infants-early introduction of lipids and use of new lipid emulsions: a systematic review. *Am J Clin Nutr*. 2012;96:255–268.
34. Driscoll DF, Nehne J, Peterss H. Physicochemical stability of intravenous lipid emulsions as all-in-one admixtures intended for the very young. *Clin Nutr.* 2003;22:489–495.
35. Athanasiou C, Hatziantoniou S, Skouroliakou M, Markantonis-Kyroudis S. Assessment of physicochemical stability of all-in-one parenteral emulsions for neonates according to USP specifications. *JPEN J Parenter Enteral Nutr*. 2014;38:867–872.
36. Rigo J, Senterre T. Intrauterine-like growth rates can be achieved with premixed parenteral nutrition solution in preterm infants. *J Nutr*. 2013;143(12 Suppl):2066S-2070S.
37. Vlaardingerbroek H, van Goudoever JB. Intravenous lipids in preterm infants: impact on laboratory and clinical outcomes and long-term consequences. *World Rev Nutr Diet*. 2015;112:71–80. doi: 10.1159/000365459.
38. Prasertsom W, Phillipos EZ, Van Aerde JE, Robertson M. Pulmonary vascular resistance during lipid in infusion in neonates. *Arch Dis Child Fetal Neonatal Ed*. 1996;74(2):F95–F98.

39. Shouman B, Abdel-Hady H, Badr RI, Hammad E, Salama MF. Dose of intravenous lipids and rate of bacterial clearance in preterm infants with blood stream infections. *Eur J Pediatr*. 2012;171(5):811–816.
40. Baumgart S, Costarino AT. Water and electrolyte metabolism of the micropremie. *Clin Perinatol.* 2000;27:131–146.
41. Ross JR, Finch C, Ebeling M, Taylor SN. Refeeding syndrome in very-low-birth-weight intrauterine growth-restricted neonates. *J Perinatol*. 2013;33:717.720.
42. Peters O, Ryan S, Matthew L, Cheng K, Lunn J. Randomised controlled trial of acetate in preterm neonates receiving parenteral nutrition. *Arch Dis Child Fetal Neonatal Ed.* 1997;77:F12–F15.
43. Aladangady N, Coen PG, White MP, Rae MD, Beattie TJ. Urinary excretion of calcium and phosphate in preterm infants. *Pediatr Nephrol.* 2004;19:1225–1231.
44. Bonsante F, Iacobelli S, Latorre G, Rigo J, De Felice C, Robillard PY, Gouyom JB. Initial amino acid intake influences phosphorus and calcium homeostasis in preterm infants: it is time to change the composition of the early parenteral nutrition. *PLoSOne.* 2013;8(8):e72880. doi: 10.1371/journal.ponc.0072880.
45. Nandivada P, Potemkin AK, Carlson SJ, Chang MI, Cowan E, O'Loughlin AA, Gura KM, Puder M. Elevated alkaline phosphatase in infants with parenteral nutrition-associated liver disease reflects bone rather than liver disease. *JPEN J Parenter Enteral Nutr.* 2014;doi:10.1177/0148607114545995.
46. Greene HL, Phillips BL. Vitamin dosages for premature infants. *Pediatrics.* 1988;81:173–174.
47. Laborie S, Lavoie JC, Chessex P. Increased urinary peroxides in newborn infants receiving parenteral nutrition exposed to light. *J Pediatr.* 2000;136:628–632.
48. Chessex P, Laborie S, Lavoie JC, Rouleau T. Photoprotection of solutions of parenteral nutrition decreases the infused load as well as the urinary excretion of peroxides in premature infants. *Semin Perinatol.* 2001;25:55–59.
49. A.S.P.E.N. position paper: recommendations for changes in commercially available parenteral multivitamin and multi-trace element products *Nutr Clin Pract.* 2012;27(4):440–491.
50. Finch CW. Review of trace element requirements for preterm infants: what are the current recommendations for clinical practice? *Nutr Clin Pract* 2015; 30(1):44–58.
51. Zambrano E, El-Hennawy M, Ehrenkranz RA, Zelterman D, Reyes-Mugica M. Total parenteral nutrition induced liver

pathology: an autopsy series of 24 newborn cases. *Pediatr Dev Pathol.* 2004;7:425–432.

52. Hurwitz M, Garcia MG, Poole RL, Kerner JA. Copper deficiency during parenteral nutrition: a report of four pediatric cases. *Nutr Clin Pract.* 2004;19:305–308.
53. Fok TF, Chui KK, Cheung R, Ng PC, Cheung KL, Hjelm M. Manganese intake and cholestatic jaundice in neonates receiving parenteral nutrition: a randomized controlled study. *Acta Paediatr.* 2001;90:1009–1015.
54. Erikson KM, Thompson K, Aschner J, Aschner M. Manganese neurotoxicity: a focus on the neonate. *Pharmacol Ther.* 2007;113:369–377.
55. Ibrahim M, Sinn J, McGuire W. Iodine supplementation for the prevention of mortality and adverse neurodevelopmental outcomes in preterm infants. *Cochrane Database Syst Rev.* 2006;(2):CD005253.
56. Ghirri P, Lunardi S, Boldrini A. Iodine supplementation in the newborn. *Nutrients.* 2014;6:382–390.
57. Soghier LM, Brion LP. Cysteine, cysteine or N-acetylcysteine supplementation in parenterally fed neonates. *Cochrane Database Syst Rev*. 2006;(4):CD004869.
58. Laine L, Shulman RJ, Pitre D, Lifschitz CH, Adams J. Cysteine usage increases the need for acetate in neonates who receive total parenteral nutrition. *Am J Clin Nutr.* 1991;54:565–567.
59. Penn D, Schmidt-Sommerfeld E, Pascu F. Decreased tissue carnitine concentrations in newborn infants receiving total parenteral nutrition. *J Pediatr.* 1981;98:976–978.
60. Cairns PA, Stalker DJ. Carnitine supplementation of parenterally fed neonates. *Cochrane Database System Rev.* 2000;(4):CD000950. doi: 10.1002/14651858.CD000950.
61. Randolph AG, Cook DJ, Gonzales CA, Andrew M. Benefit of heparin in peripheral venous and arterial catheters: systematic review and meta-analysis of randomised controlled trials. *BMJ.* 1998;316:969–975.
62. Shah P, Shah V. Continuous heparin infusion to prevent thrombosis and catheter occlusion in neonates with peripherally placed percutaneous central venous catheters. *Cochrane Database System Rev.* 2005;(3):CD002772. doi: 10.1002/14651858.CD002772.pub2.
63. Shah PS, Ng E, Sinha AK. Heparin for prolonging peripheral intravenous catheter use in neonates. *Cochrane Database System*

Rev. 2005;(4):CD002774. doi: 10.1002/14651858.CD002774.pub2.

64. Malloy MH, Cutter GR. The association of heparin exposure with intraventricular hemorrhage among very low birth weight infants. *J Perinatol.* 1995;15:185–191.
65. Ng SM, May JE, Emmerson AJ. Continuous insulin infusion in hyperglycaemic extremely-low-birth-weight neonates. *Biol Neonate.* 2005;87:269–272.
66. Alaedeen DI, Walsh MC, Chwals WJ. Total parenteral nutrition-associated hyperglycemia correlates with prolonged mechanical ventilation and hospital stay in septic infants. *J Pediatr Surg.* 2006;41:239–244.
67. Ziegler EE, Thureen PJ, Carlson SJ. Aggressive nutrition of the very low birth weight infant. *Clin Perinatol.* 2002;29:225–244.
68. Poindexter BB, Karn CA, Denne SC. Exogenous insulin reduces proteolysis and protein synthesis in extremely low birth weight infants. *J Pediatr.* 1998;132:948–953.
69. Denne SC, Poindexter BB. Evidence supporting early nutritional support with parenteral amino acid infusion. *Semin Perinatol.* 2007;31:56–60.
70. Miller M, Vaidya R, Rastogi D, Bhutada A, Rastogi S. From parenteral to enteral nutrition: a nutrition-based approach for evaluating postnatal growth failure in preterm infants. *JPEN J Parenter Enteral Nutr.* 2014;38(4):489–497.
71. Calkins KL, Venick RS, Devaskar SU. Complications associated with parenteral nutrition. *Clin Perinatol.* 2014;41:331–345.
72. Kelly DA. Intestinal failure-associated liver disease: what do we know today? *Gastroenterology.* 2006;130(2 Suppl):S70–S77.
73. Lauriti G, Zani A, Aufieri R, Cananzi M, Chiesa PL, Eaton S, Pierro A. Incidence, prevention, and treatment of parenteral nutrition-associated cholestasis and intestinal failure-associated liver disease in infants and children: a systematic review. *JPEN J Parenter Enteral Nutr.* 2014;38:70–85.
74. Shamir R, Maayan-Metzger A, Bujanover Y, Ashkenazi S, Dinari G, Sirota L. Liver enzyme abnormalities in gram-negative bacteremia of premature infants. *Pediatr Infect Dis J.* 2000;19:495–498.
75. Baserga MC, Sola A. Intrauterine growth restriction impacts tolerance to total parenteral nutrition in extremely low birth weight infants. *J Perinatol.* 2004;24:476–481.

76. Gupta K, Wang H, Amin SB. Parenteral nutrition-associated cholestasis in premature infants: role of macronutrients. *JPEN J Parenter Enteral Nutr*. 2014; doi: 10.1177/0148607114555161
77. Abrams SA. Impact of new-generation parenteral lipid emulsions in pediatric nutrition. *Adv Nutr.* 2013;4:518–520.
78. Nehra D, Fallon EM, Carlson SJ, Potemkin AK, Hevelone ND, Mitchell PD, Gura KM, Puder M. Provision of a soy-based intravenous lipid emulsion at 1 g/kg/d does not prevent cholestasis in neonates. *JPEN J Parenter Enteral Nutr*. 2013;37:498–505.
79. Levit OL, Calkins KL, Gibson LC, Kelley-Quon L et al. Low dose intravenous soybean oil emulsion for prevention of cholestasis in preterm neonates. *JPEN J Parenter Enteral Nutr.* 2014; doi: 10.1177/0148607114540005.
80. Rollins M, Ward RM, Jackson WD, Mulroy CW, Spencer CP, Ying J, Greene T, Book LS. Effect of decreased parenteral soybean lipid emulsion on hepatic function in infants at risk for parenteral nutrition-associated liver disease: A pilot study. *J Pediatr Surg*. 2013;48:1348–56.
81. Sanchez SE, Braun LP, Mercer LD, Sherrill M, Stevens J, Javid PJ. The effect of lipid restriction on the prevention of parenteral nutrition-associated cholestasis in surgical infants. *J Pediatr Surg*. 2013;48:573–578.
82. Cober MP, Killu G, Brattain A, Welch KB, Kunisaki SM, Teitelbaum DH. Intravenous fat emulsions reduction for patients with parenteral nutrition–associated liver disease. *J Pediatr*. 2012;160:421–427.
83. Thibault M, McMahon J, Faubert G, Charbonneau J, Malo J, Ferreira E, Mohamed I. Parenteral nutrition-associated liver disease: a retrospective study of ursodeoxycholic acid use in neonates. *J Pediatr Pharmacol Ther*. 2014;19(1):42–48.
84. Spencer AU, Yu S, Tracy TF, Aouthmany MM, Llanos A, Brown MB, Brown M, Shulman RJ, Hirschl RB, Derusso PA, Cox J, Dahlgren J, Strouse PJ, Groner JI, Teitelbaum DH. Parenteral nutrition-associated cholestasis in neonates: multivariate analysis of the potential protective effect of taurine. *JPEN J Parent Enteral Nutr.* 2005;29:337–343; discussion 343–344.
85. Abrams SA. Impact of new-generation parenteral lipid emulsions in pediatric nutrition. *Adv Nutr*. 2013;4:518–520.
86. Klein GL. Metabolic bone disease of total parenteral nutrition. *Nutrition.* 1998;14:149–152.

87. Backstrom MC, Kouri T, Kuusela AL, Sievanen H, Koivisto AM, Ikonen RS, Maki M. Bone isoenzyme of serum alkaline phosphatase and serum inorganic phosphate in metabolic bone disease of prematurity. *Acta Paediatr.* 2000;89:867–873.
88. Gura KM, Puder M. Recent developments in aluminium contamination of products used in parenteral nutrition. *Curr Opin Clin Nutr Metab Care.* 2006;9:239–246.
89. Young D. FDA aluminum rule poses challenges for industry, pharmacists. *Am J Health Syst Pharm.* 2004;61:742,744.
90. Kanarek KS, Kuznicki MB, Blair RC. Infusion of total parenteral nutrition via the umbilical artery. *JPEN J Parenter Enteral Nutr.* 1991;15:71–74.
91. Butler-O'Hara M, D'Angio CT, Hoey H, Stevens TP. An evidenced-based catheter bundle alters central venous catheter strategy in newborn infants. *J Pediatr*. 2012;160(6):972–977.
92. Kuwahara T, Asanami S, Tamura T, Kaneda S. Effects of pH and osmolality on phlebitic potential of infusion solutions for peripheral parenteral nutrition. *J Toxicol Sci.* 1998;23:77–85.
93. Dugan S, Le J, Jew R. Maximum tolerated osmolality for peripheral parenteral administration of parenteral nutrition in pediatric patients. *JPEN J Parenter Enteral Nutr*. 2014;38:847–851.
94. Foster J, Richards R, Showell M. Intravenous in-line filters for preventing morbidity and mortality in neonates. *Cochrane Database Syst Rev.* 2006;(2):CD005248.
95. Jack T, Boehne M, Brent BE, Hoy L, Koditz H, Wessel A, Sasse M. In-line filtration reduces severe complications and length of stay on pediatric intensive care unit: a prospective randomized controlled trial. *Intensive Care Med*. 2012;38(6):1008–1016.
96. Nghiem-Rao TH, Cassidy LD, Polzin EM, Calkins CM, Arca MJ, Goday PS. Risks and benefits of prophylactic cyclic parenteral nutrition in surgical neonates. *Nutr Clin Pract.* 2013;28:745–752.
97. Hanson C, Thoene M, Wagner J, Collier D, Lecci K, Anderson-Berry A. Parenteral nutrition additive shortages: the short-term, long-term and potential epigenetic implications in premature and hospitalized infants. *Nutrients*. 2012;4:1977–1988.
98. Mirtallo J, Holcombe B, Kochevar M, Guenter P. Parenteral nutrition product shortages: the A.S.P.E.N. strategy. *Nutr Clin Pract.* 2012;27:385–391.

Chapter 3

Enteral Nutrition

Amy Sapsford, RD, CSP, LD, CNSC, and
Carrie Smith, MS, RD, LD

OBJECTIVES

- Construct feeding plan options to maximize nutritional intake through the use of human milk, human milk fortifiers, and preterm formulas.
- Identify appropriate vitamin and mineral supplement regimens for hospitalized newborns.
- Describe enteral feeding preparation, protocols, methods, and equipment.

INTRODUCTION

Enteral nutrition (EN) is the preferred method for nourishing all infants, but for high-risk neonates it is introduced in conjunction with or when transitioning from parenteral nutrition (PN). The goal of this chapter is to provide neonatal health care professionals with evidence-based information about human milk, commercial enteral products for infants, and suggestions for introducing and progressing enteral feedings.

HUMAN MILK

Human milk is the gold standard for infant feeding and is preferred for nearly all high-risk newborns. Benefits of using human milk include improved developmental outcomes and decreased incidence of infections such as necrotizing enterocolitis (NEC) and late-onset sepsis (1–6). Box 3.1 lists conditions in which breastfeeding or human milk may be used (1,7–9). There are times when use of human milk is contraindicated (1,8,9). Families should be educated to begin breastfeeding or pumping early and use a hospital-grade pump. Many family resources are available online and are available in Spanish as well (10).

Box 3.1 Conditions Compatible with Breastfeeding or Using Human Milk

- Mothers who are hepatitis B surface antigen–positive
- Mothers infected with hepatitis A or C
- Mothers who are febrile
- Mothers exposed to low-level environmental chemical agents
- Mothers who are seropositive for cytomegalovirus (CMV)
- Mothers who smoke tobacco (mother should be advised to quit smoking)
- Mothers who drink a single, small alcoholic beverage (avoid breastfeeding or pumping for a minimum of 2 hours)
- Hyperbilirubinemia in the baby

Source: Data are from references 1, 7–9.

Storage

Human milk is stored in containers suitable for food, such as those made from polypropylene (PP), polyethylene teraphthalate (PETE), and high-density polyethylene

(HDPE) (11,12). Containers or bottles made of polycarbonate contain bisphenol A and may pose health risks (13). Some of the manufacturers that make storage containers include the following:

- Abbott Nutrition (http://abbottnutrition.com; 800/227-5767)
- Capital Vial and Snappies (www.capitalvial.com/containers/breast-milk-storage; www.snappiescontainers.com; 800/772-8871)
- Medela (www.medelabreastfeedingus.com; 800/435-8316)
- NeoMed (www.neomedinc.com; 888/876-2225)

Once expressed, human milk should be stored in a refrigerator (at 4°C or 39° to 40°F) if it will be used within the next 48 hours for hospitalized infants; otherwise it should be frozen immediately. One study showed refrigerated milk is safe stored in the refrigerator up to 96 hours in a laboratory versus clinical environment (14). The Human Milk Banking Association of North America (HMBANA) has accepted and recommends this practice (12), while some NICUs use more conservative refrigeration times for immunocompromised infants. The CDC guidelines are for healthy, term infants (15). Milk stored in a deep freezer (-20°C or -4°F) will last 6 to 12 months (11,12,16).

Thawed and fortified human milk should be used within 24 hours. Milk should not be kept at room temperature for more than 4 hours for hospitalized infants. Detailed storage guidelines for human milk are available (11,12). Some hospitals use commercial milk warmers, such as Penguin (http://crecheinnovations.com/) and the Waterless Milk Warmer (www.medelabreastfeedingus.com/for-professionals/products/516/waterless-milk-warmer)

(17,18). Hospitals should write policies and train staff to ensure proper use of these warmers. Milk may be thawed from frozen state to refrigerator temperature versus body temperature to ensure it stays in a safe temperature zone for the maximum amount of time. Likewise, milk may be warmed from refrigerator temperature to body temperature if it will be fed immediately. Milk warming practices have been reviewed (19). Milk laboratories may use commercial thawing or warming techniques.

Labeling

Guidelines have been developed for management of human milk delivery in the neonatal intensive care unit (NICU) (11,12). Human milk is labeled with two identifiers, including name and medical record number (20). The mother records the date and time the milk was expressed on the label, and nurses double-check the milk before feeding to avoid the risk of feeding an infant another mother's milk. Hospitals may do this manually or electronically with bar code systems. Regardless of how the double check is done, the nurse should always ensure the right milk is being given to the right infant. In addition, the label notes when the milk expires and whether it was fresh or frozen then thawed (11,12). Current computerized breast milk labeling systems include:

- NeoMed (http://neomedinc.com/products-safebaby.html; 888/876-2225)
- SafeBaby (http://safebabybmt.com; 800/211-0768)
- Timeless Medical Systems (www.timelessmedical.com/products/womenandinfants/#breast-milk-tracking; 800/630-3730)

Composition

Human milk composition varies throughout lactation, within a feeding, day to day, and based on the mother's diet. Macronutrient sources include lactose, whey-predominant protein, and long-chain triglycerides. For several weeks postpartum, human milk from mothers of preterm infants is known to contain greater amounts of protein and sodium than human milk from mothers of term infants (2,21). After a mother has expressed milk for one month, the protein content is inadequate to meet the needs of a preterm infant at typical fluid volumes. The docosahexaenoic acid (DHA) intake of mothers and the composition of human milk and donor human milk have been found to be low. Supplementation with a single-cell algal DHA product up to 1 g/d improved dietary DHA and maternal milk concentrations that were similar to intrauterine goals for the preterm infant (22). Human milk analyzers are available to determine macronutrient content; however, there are limitations to their use, and they are not currently approved by the FDA (23).

Donor Human Milk

Donor human milk is available for infants whose mothers are unable to express their own milk or have inadequate milk supply. Use of donor human milk may reduce the risk of NEC and is recommended in the absence of maternal breast milk for very-low-birth-weight (VLBW) infants (1,24–27). Some facilities use donor human milk as a bridge for feeding infants in the first few days of life, up to 30 days of life, or to a specific corrected gestational age (GA). Others use it when a mother wants her baby to receive only human milk but the mother's supply is inadequate.

Use of unfortified donor human milk may be associated with poor growth (24). HMBANA has established guidelines for safe and consistent handling of donor human milk (28). Donor milk can be obtained from a milk bank established through HMBANA. Prolacta (www.prolacta.com) also has a donor milk program. A new, shelf-stable donor human milk has been developed by Medolac (www.medolac.com/products--research.html); however, limited data are available for use in neonates. Use of milk obtained by purchase on the internet should be avoided (29).

HUMAN MILK FORTIFIERS AND INFANT FORMULAS

Although human milk is preferred to infant formula, for preterm infants it is inadequate in protein, many vitamins, and most minerals, including calcium, phosphorus, zinc, sodium, and iron (21). Fortifying human milk can minimize these nutrient deficiencies. Commercial bovine-based or protein hydrolysate human milk fortifiers (HMF) are available as powders and commercially sterile liquids. A human milk–based HMF is also available from Prolacta (www.prolacta.com), with literature suggesting a potential reduction in NEC rates (30). Commercial human milk fortifiers may be used up to a term baby weight of 3.5 kg and are indicated for infants who are (21):

- ≤ 34 weeks' gestation
- ≤ 1,500 g at birth
- On total parenteral nutrition > 2 weeks
- > 1,500 g at birth with suboptimal growth
- > 1,500 g at birth with limited ability to tolerate increased volume

The addition of powdered and liquid HMF to expressed human milk increases the osmolality. Tolerance may be improved by starting with 1 packet of HMF mixed with 50 mL of expressed human milk (22 kcal/oz) and progressing to 1 packet to 25 mL (24 kcal/oz) as tolerated and according to manufacturers' directions.

For babies whose mothers choose not to provide human milk or for when the supply of human milk is exhausted, commercial infant formulas designed for preterm infants are available and highly recommended (21,31,32). Preterm infants fed formulas designed for preterm infants have better growth, nitrogen retention, and bone mineral content than preterm infants fed standard formulas (21).

A variety of soy, protein hydrolysate, and amino acid–based formulas are available when preterm infants do not tolerate preterm infant formulas. Although satisfactory for term infants, these products may not be nutritionally adequate for growing preterm infants when fed at 20 kcal/oz. Soy protein–based formulas are specifically not recommended for preterm infants (33–35). Preterm infants not on fortified human milk or a commercial preterm formula should be closely monitored and considered for enrichment with modular products (refer to Box 3.2) and/or vitamin/mineral supplements. A summary of selected multivitamin and mineral supplements for children has been published (36). A gradual transition back to fortified human milk or preterm formula is suggested if the baby's condition allows it. See Box 3.3 and Table 3.1 for more information.

Box 3.2 Modular Products

Protein

- Abbott Nutrition Liquid Protein Fortifier, Nutricia Complete Amino Acids, Nestle Beneprotein[a]
- Common sources are whey protein isolate or amino acids.
- Typically, powdered protein supplements provide 0.8–0.9 g protein and 3.2–3.6 kcal per gram of powder.
- Typically powdered protein supplements provide 7 g powder/scoop, 4.7 or 9.5 g powder/Tbsp.
- Liquid protein fortifier provides 1 g protein (extensively hydrolyzed casein) and 4 kcal per 6 mL liquid; 0.17g protein and 0.67 kcal per mL. This supplement has the added benefit of being sterile.

Carbohydrate

- Nutricia Polycal Powder
- Common source is polysaccharides.
- Per 5 g of powder, provides 4.8 g carbohydrates, 19 kcal.

Fat

- Nestle Nutrition Microlipid, MCT oil, vegetable oils
- Common sources are coconut oil, 100% safflower oil, and vegetable/corn oils. Microlipid is emulsified.
- Provide 0.5–1 g fat (4.5–8 kcal) per mL.

Carbohydrate and fat

- Nutricia Duocal
- Provides 4.9 kcal (0.73 g carbohydrates as hydrolyzed corn starch, 0.22 g fat as corn/coconut/MCT oil) per gram of powder.
- Provides 5 g powder per scoop, 8.5 g powder/Tbsp

Note: Powdered supplements are not commercially sterile and should not be used in the NICU setting or in infants who are immunocompromised, unless there is no nutritionally appropriate alternative available.

[a] Appropriate for use in children greater than 3 years of age but is known to be used in infants (37).

Box 3.3 Human Milk, Human Milk Fortifiers, and Infant Formulas: Availability, Indications, and Macronutrient Sources

Human milk (Maternal breast milk or donor milk)

- From mothers who wish to breastfeed or who pump to provide expressed milk; from human milk banks
- **Indications:** Preterm infants; infants birth to 1 year and beyond; donor milk for use when maternal breast milk is not available—strongest indication for VLBW infants
- **Carbohydrate:** Lactose
- **Protein:** Human milk
- **Fat:** LCT Human milk

Human milk fortifiers

- Bovine powder, liquid
  - **Examples:** Enfamil[a] (HMF powder, HMF acidified liquid), Similac[b] (HMF powder, HMF concentrated liquid, HMF hydrolyzed protein concentrated liquid)
- Human milk–based liquid
  - **Examples:** Prolact+H[2]MF[c]
- **Indications:** Multinutrient supplement to be added to human milk to meet nutrition needs for premature or low birth weight infants
- **Carbohydrate:** Corn syrup solids; maltodextrin (liquid only); lactose (human milk–based)
- **Protein:** Cow's milk protein (bovine based) (intact, whey protein isolate, and hydrolyzed); human milk protein (human milk based)
- **Fat:** Variety of vegetable oils and/or MCT (70%–100%) (bovine based); LCT (human milk based)

(continued)

Box 3.3 Human Milk, Human Milk Fortifiers, and Infant Formulas: Availability, Indications, and Macronutrient Sources (continued)

Preterm formulas

- Ready-to-feed liquid in a variety of caloric densities and protein content
- **Examples:** Enfamil Premature[a], Gerber Good Start Premature[d], Similac Special Care[b]
- **Indications:** Contain higher amounts of nutrients including protein, vitamins, and minerals to meet the needs of growing premature infants; suitable for use as HMF
- **Carbohydrate:** Corn syrup solids or maltodextrin, and lactose (50%)
- **Protein:** Cow's milk protein (intact and partially hydrolyzed)
- **Fat:** Variety of vegetable oils and MCT (40%–50%)

Preterm discharge formulas

- Ready-to-feed liquid; powder
- **Examples:** Enfamil EnfaCare[a], Similac Expert Care NeoSure[b]
- **Indications:** For the continued feeding of preterm infants with nutrient density between preterm and most standard milk protein–based formulas
- **Carbohydrate:** Corn syrup solids or maltodextrin, and lactose (40%–70%)
- **Protein:** Cow's milk protein (intact)
- **Fat:** Variety of vegetable oils and MCT (20%–25%)

Standard milk protein–based formulas

- Ready-to-feed liquid; liquid concentrate; powder
- **Examples:** Enfamil Newborn[a], Enfamil Infant[a], Gerber Good Start Gentle[d], Similac Advance[b]
- **Indications:** Infants birth to 1 year
- **Carbohydrate:** Lactose, corn maltodextrin
- **Protein:** Cow's milk protein (intact and partially hydrolyzed)
- **Fat:** Variety of vegetable oils

(continued)

Box 3.3 Human Milk, Human Milk Fortifiers, and Infant Formulas: Availability, Indications, and Macronutrient Sources (continued)

Soy protein–based formulas

- Ready-to-feed liquid; liquid concentrate; powder
- **Examples:** Enfamil ProSobee[a], Gerber Good Start Soy[d], Similac Soy Isomil[b]
- **Indications:** Infants birth to 1 year with IgE-mediated allergy or sensitivity to cow milk protein; lactose-free for disorders such as galactosemia or congenital lactase deficiency (rare). (Note: Should be used with caution in preterm infants.)
- **Carbohydrate:** Corn syrup solids, corn maltodextrin, sucrose ranging from 0%–40%
- **Protein:** Soy protein isolate, L-methionine
- **Fat:** Variety of vegetable oils

Tolerance formulas

- Ready-to-feed; powder
- **Examples:** Enfamil Gentlease[a], Enfamil Reguline[a], Gerber Good Start Soothe[d], Similac Sensitive[b], Similac Total Comfort[b]
- **Indications:** Extreme fussiness, gas; withdrawal (See Chapter 16 Neonatal Abstinence Syndrome)
- **Carbohydrate:** Corn syrup solids, corn maltodextrin, prebiotics/probiotics, sucrose, lactose ranging from 0%–50%
- **Protein:** Cow's milk protein (partially hydrolyzed and/or intact)
- **Fat:** Variety of vegetable oils

Semielemental formulas

- Liquid concentrate and/or ready-to-feed liquid; powder
- **Examples:** Enfamil Nutramigen[a], Enfamil Pregestimil[a], Similac Expert Care Alimentum[b]
- **Indications:** Hypoallergenic formula for infants birth to 1 year sensitive to intact protein found in milk- and soy-based formulas
- **Carbohydrate:** Variety of sources (lactose-free)
- **Protein:** Casein hydrolysate, L-cystine, L-tyrosine, and L-tryptophan
- **Fat:** Variety of vegetable oils, MCT (0%–55%)

(continued)

Box 3.3 Human Milk, Human Milk Fortifiers, and Infant Formulas: Availability, Indications, and Macronutrient Sources (continued)

Elemental formulas

- Powder (Note: Product is *not* packaged ready-to-use.)
- **Examples:** PurAmino[a], EleCare[b], Neocate[e]
- **Indications:** Amino acid–based formula for infants and young children with severe allergy to intact protein
- **Carbohydrate:** Corn syrup solids and/or modified corn starch
- **Protein:** Free amino acids
- **Fat:** Variety of vegetable oils, MCT (0%–33%)

Source: Data are from references 33 and 35.

Abbreviations: IgE, immunoglobulin E; LBW, low birth weight; LCT, long-chain triglycerides; MCT, medium-chain triglycerides; HMF, human milk fortifier.

[a]Mead Johnson (www.meadjohnson.com/pediatrics/us-en)

[b]Abbott (www.abbottnutrition.com)

[c]Prolacta BioScience (www.prolacta.com)

[d]Gerber (www.medical.gerber.com)

[e]Nutricia (www.neocate.com)

Note: Product information is subject to change. Please consult manufacturer websites, product handbooks, and product labels for specific information on ingredients.

Table 3.1 Typical Value Ranges for Selected Nutrients in Human Milk, Human Milk Fortifiers, and Infant Formulas

	Energy, kcal/dL	Protein, g/dL	Sodium, mg/dL (mEq/dL)	Calcium, mg/dL	Phosphorus, mg/dL	Osmolality, mOsm/kg H_20
Human milk, term[a]	70	0.9	18 (0.8)	28	15	290
Human milk, preterm	67	1.4	25 (1.1)	25	13	290
HMF: Composition for 4 packets of powder	14–15	1.0–1.1	15–16 (0.7)	90–117	50–67	—
HMF: Composition for 4 packets of concentrated liquid	14	1.4–2.2	20–27 (0.8–1.2)	120–140	68–80	—
HMF (powder) mixed with preterm human milk (1 packet per 25 mL)	79	2.4–2.5	39–41 (1.7–1.9)	115–138	63–78	325–385
HMF (liquid) mixed with preterm human milk (1 packet per 25 mL)	79	2.8–3.6	45–52 (1.9–2.3)	140–175	75–90	325–450
Preterm formulas: 20 kcal/oz	68	2	29–39 (1.3–1.7)	111–122	56–68	220–235
Preterm formulas: 24 kcal/oz	81	2.4–2.9	35–47 (1.5–2)	133–146	67–81	280–300

Preterm formulas: 30 kcal/oz	101	3	44–59 (1.9–2.6)	167–183	84–101	320–341
Preterm discharge formulas	73–74	2–2.1	25–27 (1.1–1.2)	78–89	46–49	250–310
Milk protein–based formulas	64	1.3–1.5	16–18 (0.7–0.8)	45–53	26–28	250–310
Soy protein–based formulas	64–68	1.6–1.7	27–30 (1.2–1.3)	71	43–52	170–200
Tolerance formulas	64–68	1.4–1.5	18–30 (0.8–1.3)	49–68	27–45	195–230
Semi-elemental formulas	54–68	1.9	29–32 (1.3–1.4)	63–71	35–51	260–370
Elemental formulas	68	1.9–2.1	25–32 (1.1–1.4)	63–83	42–62	350–375

Abbreviation: HMF, human milk fortifier.

Note: Product information varies. Please consult manufacturer websites, product handbooks, and specific product labels for information on nutrients and osmolality.

Source: Term human milk data in row 1 are from reference 7. Preterm human milk composition summary is from Abbott Nutrition (Columbus, OH).

ENTERAL NUTRIENT REQUIREMENTS

Enteral nutrient requirements for infants vary by body weight and age. Preterm infant needs are greater than those of term infants due to decreased nutrient stores, altered gastrointestinal absorption, diseases or conditions, and rapid rates of weight gain. Nutrients of particular interest in the preterm infant include protein, calcium, iron, phosphorus, sodium, vitamin D, and zinc. Recommended intakes for most nutrients can typically be achieved by feeding fortified human milk or high-protein premature formulas. Vitamin and mineral supplements and/or modular macronutrient products are needed when commercially available formulas do not meet the needs of the infant. Standard of care for enteral nutrient requirements for preterm infants was formerly derived from data by Tsang and colleagues (38). Those recommendations were recently revised by Koletzko and colleagues (39). In addition, recommendations for enteral intakes for stable preterm infants up to a weight of approximately 1,800 grams are available from the Committee on Nutrition of the European Society of Paediatric Gastroenterology, Hepatology, and Nutrition (ESPGHAN) (40). In practice, clinicians use recommendations for VLBW infants up to approximately term infant age and weight and then transition to the Recommended Dietary Allowances and Adequate Intakes (RDAs and AIs) (see Tables 3.2–3.5) (38–41).

Table 3.2 Enteral Nutrient Requirements for Fully Enterally Fed Preterm VLBW Infants (< 1,500 g): Fluids, Energy, and Macronutrients

Nutrient	Koletzko, et al 2014	ESPGHAN, 2010	RDA/AI[a] (Age 0–6 mo)
Fluid	135–200 mL/kg[b]	135–200 mL/kg	0.7 L/d
Energy	110–130 kcal/kg[c]	110–135 kcal/kg	555/d
Carbohydrate	11.6–13.2 g/kg[c]	11.6–13.2 g/kg	60 g/d
Protein	3.5–4.5 g/kg[c]	4–4.5 (< 1 kg) 3.5–4 (1–1.8 kg)	9.1 g/d
Fat	4.8–6.6 g/kg	4.8–6.6 g/kg (40% MCT)	31 g/d
Linoleic acid	385–1540 mg/kg	385–1540 mg/kg	4.4 g/d (14%)
α-Linolenic acid	> 55 mg/kg	> 55 mg/kg	0.5 g/d (1.6%)
DHA	55–60 mg/kg	12–30 mg/kg	—
AA	35–45 mg/kg	18–42 mg/kg	—

Abbreviations: DHA, docosahexaenoic acid; AA, arachidonic acid; VLBW, very low birth weight; RDA, Recommended Dietary Allowance; AI, Adequate Intake.

[a]Recommended Dietary Allowances (RDAs) and Adequate Intakes (AIs) may both be used as goals for individual intake. RDAs are set to meet the needs of almost all (97%–98%) individuals in a group. For healthy infants fed human milk, the AI is the mean intake (41).

[b]New recommendations are essentially the same as Tsang 2005 (38).

[c]New recommendations are essentially higher than Tsang 2005 (38).

Source: Data are from references 38–41.

Table 3.3 Enteral Nutrient Requirements for Fully Enterally Fed Preterm VLBW Infants: Minerals

Mineral	Koletzko, et al 2014	ESPGHAN, 2010	RDA/AI[a] (Age 0–6 mo)
Calcium	120–200 mg/kg[b]	120–140 mg/kg	210 mg/d
Phosphorus	60–140 mg/kg[c]	60–90 mg/kg	100 mg/d
Magnesium	8–15 mg/kg[c]	8–15 mg/kg	30 mg/d
Sodium	3–5 mEq/kg (69–115 mg/kg)[d]	3–5 mEq/kg (69–115 mg/kg)	120 mg/d
Potassium	2–5 mEq/kg (78–195 mg/kg)[d]	1.7–3.4 mEq/kg (66–132 mg/kg)	400 mg/d
Chloride	3–5 mEq/kg (105–177 mg/kg)[d]	3–5 mEq/kg (105–177 mg/kg)	180 mg/d

Abbreviations: AI, Adequate Intake; VLBW, very low birth weight.

[a]For healthy infants fed human milk, the AI is the mean intake. All values in final two columns of this table are AIs (41).

[b]New recommendations are essentially lower than Tsang 2005 (38).

[c]New recommendations are essentially the same as Tsang 2005 (38).

[d]New recommendations are essentially higher than Tsang 2005 (38).

Source: Data are from references 38–41.

Table 3.4 Enteral Nutrient Requirements for Fully Enterally Fed Preterm VLBW Infants: Trace Elements

Trace Element	Koletzko, et al 2014[a]	ESPGHAN, 2010	RDA/AI[b] (Age 0–6 mo)
Zinc	1.4–2.5 mg/kg	1.1–2 mg/kg	2 mg/d
Copper	100–230 mcg/kg	100–132 mcg/kg	200 mcg/d
Iron	2–3 mg/kg	2–3 mg/kg	0.27 mg/d
Chromium	30–2250 ng/kg	30–1230 ng/kg	0.2 mcg/d
Molybdenum	0.3–5 mcg/kg	0.3–5 mcg/kg	2 mcg/d
Manganese	1–15 mcg/kg	< 27.5 mcg/kg	0.003 mg/d
Iodine	10–55 mcg/kg	11–55 mcg/kg	110 mcg/d
Fluoride	1.5–60 mcg/kg	1.5–60 mcg/kg	0.01 mg/d
Selenium	5–10 mcg/kg	5–10 mcg/kg	15 mcg/d

Abbreviations: RDA, Recommended Dietary Allowance; AI, Adequate Intake; ELBW, extremely low birth weight; VLBW, very low birth weight.

[a]All new recommendations are essentially higher than Tsang 2005 (38).

[b]Recommended Dietary Allowances (RDAs) and Adequate Intakes (AIs) may both be used as goals for individual intake. RDAs are set to meet the needs of almost all (97%–98%) individuals in a group. For healthy infants fed human milk, the AI is the mean intake (41).

Source: Data are from references 38–41.

Table 3.5 Enteral Nutrient Requirements for Fully Enterally Fed Preterm VLBW Infants: Vitamins

Vitamins	Koletzko, et al 2014	ESPGHAN, 2010	RDA/AI[a] (Age 0–6 mo)
Vitamin A, RE	400–1100 mcg/kg[b]	400–1100 mcg/kg	400 mcg/d[d]
Vitamin D	400–1000 IU/d (from milk + supplement)[b]	800–1000 IU/d (100–350 IU/d from milk only	5 mcg/d[e]
Vitamin E α–TE	2.2–11 mg/kg[c]	2.2–11 mg/kg	4 mg/d[f]
Vitamin K_1	4.4–28 mcg/kg	4.4–28 mcg/kg	2 mcg/d
L–Ascorbic Acid	20–55 mg/kg[b]	11–46 mg/kg	40 mg/d
Thiamin	140–300 mcg/kg[c]	140–300 mcg/kg	0.2 mg/d
Riboflavin	200–400 mcg/kg[b]	200–400 mcg/kg	0.3 mg/d
Niacin	1–5.5 mg/kg[b]	0.38–5.5 mg/kg	2 mg/d
Pyridoxine	50–300 mcg/kg[b]	45–300 mcg/kg	0.1 mg/d
Cobalamin	0.1–0.8 mcg/kg[b]	0.1–0.77 mcg/kg	0.4 mcg/d
Folic acid	35–100 mcg/kg[b]	35–100 mcg/kg	65 mcg/d
Pantothenic acid	0.5–2.1 mg/kg[b]	0.33–2.1 mg/kg	1.7 mg/d
Biotin	1.7–16.5 mcg/kg[b]	1.7–16.5 mcg/kg	5 mcg/d
Choline	8–55 mg/kg[b]	8–55 mg/kg	125 mg/d

Abbreviations: AI, Adequate Intake; RE, retinol equivalent; VLBW, very low birth weight.

[a]For healthy infants fed human milk, the AI is the mean intake. All values in final two columns of this table are AIs (41).

[b]New recommendations are essentially higher than Tsang 2005 (38).

[c]New recommendations are essentially the same as Tsang 2005 (38).

[d]New recommendations are essentially lower than Tsang 2005 (38).

[d]As retinol activity equivalents (RAEs). 1 RAE = 1 mcg retinol, 12 mcg beta carotene.

[e]As cholecalciferol. 1 mcg = 40 IU vitamin D.

[f]As alpha tocopherol.

Source: Data are from references 38–41.

Additional Nutrient Supplementation

Preterm, VLBW infants fed fortified human milk or preterm infant formulas may need additional vitamin or mineral supplementation. Current nutrient intake recommendations should be compared with actual intakes to determine if individual supplements are needed. The neonatal dietitian should be proactive in ensuring nutrient needs are being met. Products may be reformulated as nutrient recommendations change.

A nutrient of concern is vitamin D, as recommendations have significantly increased (39,42,43). With the new recommendation for vitamin D intake for preterm infants increasing up to 1,000 IU, formula and human milk–fed infants both will require supplementation. Human milk contains negligible amounts of vitamin D. Both fortified human milk and preterm infant formulas provide about 120 IU/dL vitamin D. There are no specific recommendations for monitoring 25(OH)D in preterm infants. Checking levels should be considered, especially if intake is inadequate or there are other risk factors, such as long-term TPN.

Iron stores are low for preterm infants and they lose iron from multiple blood draws. When an infant is transfused with packed red blood cells, the infant receives 1 mg elemental iron per mL blood transfused (1). The American Academy of Pediatrics (AAP) recommends iron supplementation after 2 weeks of life, assuming the infant is enterally fed, while others recommend supplementing after 2 to 6 weeks (1,39). There is no contraindication for using iron-fortified formula in a preterm infant (1). Iron supplementation should be continued after discharge. Ready-to-feed formula and most bottled water do not contain fluoride; if formula is not reconstituted with fluoridated water or sufficient fluoridated water is not consumed in some other way, a fluoride supplement of 0.25 mg/d after 6 months is recommended (1). Most hospitalized infants do not receive fluoride. If a 6-month-old baby is in the NICU, supplementation should be considered. See Boxes 3.4 and 3.5 for types of vitamin, mineral, and multivitamin supplements and manufacturer information. Also refer to a published summary of vitamin supplements (36).

Box 3.4 Selected Available Enteral Nutrition Vitamin and Mineral Supplements

Vitamins

- Vitamin A (retinol) (IM parenteral injection) Aquasol A: 50,000 units/mL
- Vitamin A generic (oral): 10,000 units/capsule
- Vitamin B-6 (pyridoxine HCl) (injection): 100 mg/mL
- Vitamin B-6 (pyridoxine HCl): 25-mg oral tablets
- Vitamin B-12 Rubimin (cyanocobalamin) (injection): 1,000 mcg/mL
- Vitamin B-12 tablet (cyanocobalamin): 50-mcg oral tablets
- Vitamin B-12 Nascobal (cyanocobalamin): 500 mcg/0.1 mL nasal spray
- Vitamin C (ascorbic acid) (drops): 500 mg/5mL oral syrup
- Vitamin C (ascorbic acid): 250-mg oral tablets
- Vitamin D D-Vi-Sol (cholecalciferol) D3: 400 IU/1 mL oral
- Vitamin D Baby Ddrops (cholecalciferol) D3: 400 IU/drop oral
- Vitamin D Bio-D-Mulsion (cholecalciferol) D3: 400 IU/drop oral
- Vitamin D (cholecalciferol) D3: 5,000–50,000 IU/capsule oral
- Vitamin D Drisdol (ergocalciferol) D2: 8,000 IU/mL oral or 200 IU/drop
- Vitamin D-2 (ergocalciferol) D2: 50,000 IU/capsule oral

(continued)

Box 3.4 Selected Available Enteral Nutrition Vitamin and Mineral Supplements (continued)

Vitamins (continued)

- Vitamin E Liqui-E TPGS (d-alpha tocopherol) 400 IU/15 mL
- Vitamin E Aquasol E: 15 IU/0.3 mL oral
- Vitamin K-1 Aqua Mephyton (phytonadione) (IV or IM): 1 mg/mL
- Vitamin K Mephyton (phytonadione): 5-mg oral tablet

Minerals

- Iron Fer-in-sol (Ferrous Sulfate) 75 mg ferrous sulfate = 15 mg elemental iron, 15 mg/mL oral drops
- Multivitamin with Iron: 10 mg/1mL (Does not contain B12 or folate)
- Iron Dextran Complex Infed: IV infusion in desired dose
- Fluoride Luride (sodium fluoride): 1.1 mg or 0.5 mg elemental fluoride/mL
- Fluoride Fluor A Day (sodium fluoride): 0.55 mg or 0.25 mg elemental fluoride/chewable tab
- Calcium calcionate: as calcium glubionate (syrup) 115.2 mg elemental calcium/5mL
- Calcium carbonate: 500 mg/5mL elemental suspension (1,250 mg calcium carbonate = 500 mg elemental calcium)
- Calcium carbonate 500 mg and Vitamin D cholecalciferol 400 IU per 5 mL oral liquid
- Magnesium sulfate (IV source used orally): 1 g of magnesium sulfate = 98.6 mg elemental magnesium = 8.12 mEq magnesium 40 mg/mL
- Magnesium sulfate oral solution: 400 mg magnesium sulfate = 40 mg elemental Mg/mL
- Sodium chloride: 2.5 mEq/mL oral solution (use salt with caution)
- Sodium Phosphate: 3 mM phosphate and 4 mEq Sodium/1 mL oral solution
- Potassium chloride Kayciel: 20 mEq/15 mL (10%) oral solution
- Potassium phosphate KPhos: 93 mg elemental phosphorus = 3mM phosphate: 4.4 mEq potassium/1 mL oral solution

(continued)

Box 3.4 Selected Available Enteral Nutrition Vitamin and Mineral Supplements (continued)

Minerals (continued)

- Sodium citrate BiCitra: 1 mL–1 mEq bicarbonate and 1 mEq sodium oral solution
- Potassium and sodium citrate PolyCitra: 1 mL oral solution contains 2 mEq bicarbonate, 1 mEq sodium, and 1 mEq potassium.
- Zinc Sulfate Heptahydrate: 8.1 mg/mL elemental zinc oral syrup

Tri–vitamins (drops, with and without iron)

- Each 1 mL typically contains 750–1,500 IU vitamin A, 35 mg vitamin C, 400 IU vitamin D; up to 10 mg iron (for multivitamins that specify "with iron")
- Lactose-free, gluten-free, no artificial sweeteners (Note: vitamin A content was decreased from 1,500 to 750 IU per mL in Tri-Vi-Sol products in 2013.)

Multivitamins (drops, with or without iron)

- Each 1 mL typically contains 750–1,500 IU vitamin A, 35 mg vitamin C, 400 IU vitamin D, 5 IU vitamin E, 0.5 mg thiamin, 0.6 mg riboflavin, 8 mg niacin, 0.4 mg vitamin B-6, 2 mcg vitamin B-12, and 10 mg iron (for multivitamins that specify "with iron"). There is no B-12 in products with iron; no folate in any product.
- Available as lactose-free, gluten-free, with no artificial sweeteners. (Note: Vitamin A content was decreased from 1,500 to 750 IU per ml in Poly-Vi-Sol products in 2013.)

Multivitamins with water-miscible formulation of fat-soluble vitamins (drops) (AquADEKs)

- Contains 5,751 IU vitamin A (87% as beta carotene); 45 mg vitamin C; 400 IU vitamin D3; 50 IU vitamin E; 400 mcg vitamin K; 0.6 mg thiamin; 0.6 mg riboflavin; 6 mg niacin; 0.6 mg vitamin B-6; 15 mcg biotin; 3 mg pantothenic acid; 5 mg zinc, 10 mcg selenium; and 2 mg Coenzyme Q10

Box 3.5 Selected Manufacturers of Brand Name Nutrient Supplements

- AquADEK Actavis Pharma (www.actavis.com)
- Aquamephyton (www.rxwiki.com/aquamephyton)
- Aquasol E Hospira (www.hospira.com)
- Biotics (http://bioticsnw.com/content/bio-d-mulsion%C2%AE-1-oz-1007)
- CalQuick (www.twinlab.com/product/cal–quick%C2%AE)
- Cobalamin (www.nascobal.com/)
- Ddrops Company (www.ddropscompany.com)
- Drisdol Ergocalciferol (www.empr.com/drisdol/drug/3865/)
- Drisdol Sanofi–Aventis (www.sanofi–aventis.us)
- Enfamil (www.enfamil.com)
- Iron Dextran (www.infed.com/)
- Luride (www.onlinedrugtest.info/generic–luride–information.html)
- Mead Johnson (www.meadjohnson.com)
- NanoVits Solace Nutrition (www.solacenutrition.com)
- Vitamin E TPGS (www.tpgs.com)

MANAGEMENT OF ENTERAL FEEDING

Feeding Methodology

Although breastfeeding or bottle feeding is the ultimate goal for high-risk newborns, most infants begin and progress to their nutrition goals by tube feeding. Feeding tubes should be:

- Radio-opaque for visualization on radiography
- Made of either polyurethane or silicone (indwelling for up to 30 days) or polyvinylchloride (for intermittent feedings; cannot be left in place)
- > 5 French (Fr) in size but < 8 Fr for satisfactory flow

Products containing the plasticizer di (2-ethylhexyl) phthalate (DEHP) are not recommended (44). Nasogastric and orogastric tube feedings are commonly used for preterm infants with feedings delivered either continuously or intermittently (bolus). Less commonly used are transpyloric (nasoduodenal and nasojejunal), jejunal, or gastrostomy feedings. Box 3.6 reviews considerations when choosing among feeding methods (1,45–48).

Box 3.6 Review of Enteral Feeding Methodologies

Gastric bolus (NG or OG)[a]

Indications:

- Premature
- Immature oral motor skills

Contraindications:

- Placement by inexperienced personnel
- NG/OG tubes are not indicated for long-term use; should not be used if a feeding tube is needed for longer than 1–2 months postdischarge.

Advantages:

- Simple
- Minimal equipment
- Initiation of feedings for infants unable to orally feed
- Minimize TPN
- Can be done at home after successful parent teaching

Disadvantages:

- Possible inability to protect airway such as absent gag reflex or aspiration

Potential problems:

- Malabsorption
- Dumping syndrome
- Aspiration
- Emesis
- Tube misplacement or dislodgement
- Nasal erosion (NG)
- Palatal grooves (OG)
- Bradycardia due to vagal stimulation

(continued)

Box 3.6 Review of Enteral Feeding Methodologies(continued)

Gastric Continuous (NG or OG)[a]

Indications:

- Malabsorption
- Reflux
- Aspiration

Contraindications:

- Same as for bolus
- Proximal ostomy
- NG/OG tubes are not indicated for long-term use; should not be used if a feeding tube is needed for longer than 1–2 months postdischarge.

Advantages:

- Well-tolerated
- Alternative to bolus feedings
- Increased absorption for infant with intestinal disease

Disadvantages:

- Same as for bolus
- Fat loss from human milk due to separation and adherence to the plastic

Potential problems:

- Pump malfunction
- Antireflux system should be considered
- Aspiration potential if tube is pulled into esophagus
- Decreased cyclic enteric hormone response

ND or NJ

Indications:

- Feeding intolerance of bolus feeds without ileus
- Severe gastroesophageal reflux

Contraindications:

- Unsafe for bolus feeding
- Placement by inexperienced personnel
- Home use
- Proximal ostomy

Advantages:

- Typically well-tolerated
- Alternative when gastric feeds not tolerated
- Less risk of aspiration

(continued)

Box 3.6 Review of Enteral Feeding Methodologies (continued)

ND or NJ (continued)

Disadvantages:

- Must always be continuous feeding

Potential problems:

- Perforation
- Dumping syndrome
- Diarrhea
- Pump malfunction
- Decreased cyclic enteric hormone response

G tube

Indications:

- Anatomical malformations
- Neurological damage
- Severe feeding aversion
- Need for long-term tube feeding (> 2–3 mo postdischarge)

Contraindications:

- Potential for full nipple feedings in a short time (1–2 mo postdischarge)
- Poor wound healing

Advantages:

- Allows for easier care at home
- Less feeding aversion than with long-term nasoenteric tube
- Safer for continuous feeding at home

Disadvantages:

- Surgical procedure

Potential problems:

- Tube displacement causing gastric outlet obstruction
- Site infections
- Leaking at the site

Jejunal (J tube)

Indications:

- Infant not able to be fed into the stomach requiring long-term access (greater than 1–2 months postdischarge)

Contraindications:

- Proximal ostomy
- Rarely used in neonates

(continued)

Box 3.6 Review of Enteral Feeding Methodologies (continued)

Jejunal (J tube) (continued)

Advantages:

- Well tolerated if access can be maintained
- Alternative method for infant not able to be fed otherwise

Disadvantages:

- Can be difficult to maintain access
- Use by inexperienced personnel
- Must always be continuous feeding

Potential problems:

- Unable to maintain access
- Perforation of the bowel wall
- Diarrhea
- Dumping syndrome, especially with hyperosmolar feeds

Abbreviations: NG, nasogastric; OG orogastric; TPN, total parenteral nutrition; ND, nasoduodenal; NJ, nasojejunal; G tube, gastrostomy tube.
Source: Data are from references 1 and 45–48.

Patient Safety

The Joint Commission issued a Sentinel Event Alert regarding tubing misconnections in 2006 that was updated in 2014 (49). Among the other misconnections, IV feeding infusions have been connected to nasogastric (NG) tubes and enteral feedings have been administered into IV lines and tracheostomy tubes (49–51). Risk-reduction strategies suggested by the Joint Commission and initiated by the International Standardization Organization are under way. They include design of the systems to be incompatible, and reengineering work practices (49,51,52). The implementation process of an enteral-only system in a NICU for nutrition and medications has been described (53).

Feeding Initiation and Advancement

When medically appropriate, enteral feedings are initiated soon after birth (1,39). Low-volume feedings of £ 20 mL/kg/d (called minimal enteral nutrition [MEN], gut stimulation, or priming feedings, trophic feedings, or hypocaloric feedings) are continued for 3 to 5 days for ELBW and sick VLBW infants. MEN can be full-strength expressed human milk or half- or full-strength preterm formula and fed either continuously or intermittently. Infants < 750 g with slow motility may benefit from MEN for a minimum of a week (54). Feedings are advanced at £ 20 to 35 mL/kg/d, depending on the size of the infant and severity of illness (25,54). Infants have been safely fed despite the presence of umbilical lines (55); however, each infant must be assessed by the attending physician. In addition, caution is recommended when beginning feedings in severely asphyxiated infants (pH < 7.1) with poor perfusion and when pressors (ie, dopamine, dobutamine) are used. A sample feeding plan is included in Box 3.7.

Early enteral feedings and a standardized approach to feeding have been shown to improve intestinal motility, stimulate hormonal response, improve feeding tolerance, promote earlier achievement of full feeds, improve growth, and decrease problems related to prolonged PN in the VLBW infant (1,39,55). There is no strong evidence that routine checking of gastric residuals in infants provides any benefit (56).

Box 3.7 Sample Feeding Plan: Cincinnati Perinatal Institute Enteral Feeding Guidelines for Infants ≤ 1,500 g

- Use of mother's own milk (MOM) is preferred.
- Ordering provider should consent guardian for donor human milk (DHM) during first conversation even if mother plans to provide milk. DHM may be used as a bridge if MOM is not available.
- If MOM is not available and guardian did not consent to use of DHM, 24 cal/oz Similac Special Care High Protein should be used.
- Begin feedings within 48 hours of life unless the baby is not hemodynamically stable.
- TPN is started in the first day of life and optimized daily as fluid needs and access allows.
- Day of Feedings 1–3: Feed 15 mL/kg/d (trophic or MEN) intermittent bolus nasogastric (NG) every 3 hours rounded to the nearest 1 mL. SGA baby may take feeds by mouth.
- Day of Feedings 4–6: Feed additional 20 mL/kg/d intermittent bolus ng divided into 2 volume changes per day (10 mL/kg/d at noon and midnight) up to 75 mL/kg/day.
- Day of Feeding 7: Hold feeds at 75 mL/kg/d and fortify to 22 al/oz with Similac Human Milk Fortifier (Hydrolysate).
- Day of Feeding 8: Hold feeds at 75 mL/kg/d and fortify to 24 cal/oz with Similac Human Milk Fortifier (Hydrolysate).
- Day of Feedings 9–13: Continue progressing by 20 mL/kg/d divided in 2 volume changes per day to a goal of 160 mL/kg/d.
- Feeding volumes are calculated based on birth weight but total fluid volume goal can be reassessed after the first week of life, which may allow for additional TPN volume. TPN should be continued as long as possible to optimize nutrition.

Abbreviations: MOM, mother's own milk; DHM, donor human milk; MEN, minimal enteral nutrition; SGA, small for gestational age; TPN, total parenteral nutrition.

Source: Copyright ©2015 Cincinnati Children's Hospital Medical Center, Cincinnati, OH. All Rights Reserved. Used with permission.

Feeding intolerance signs to monitor during enteral nutrition advancement include (57):

- Bloody stools and/or emesis
- Bilious emesis
- Increased number of apneic and/or bradycardic episodes, especially associated around feeding times
- Temperature instability
- Abdominal changes:
  - Significant increases in girth measurements
  - Noticeable loops of bowel
  - Discoloration of the skin on or around the abdomen
  - Hypoactive or hyperactive bowel sounds
  - Guarding with palpation

Transition to Oral Feeding

In addition to knowing *what* is fed, the neonatal dietitian is knowledgeable about *how* the baby is fed. The neonatal dietitian works closely with the feeding experts in the NICU, including nurses and speech and occupational therapists. Many infants benefit from tastes of human milk or formula via pacifier in preparation for oral feedings of larger volume. Skin-to-skin contact is beneficial for all babies, including those who will be nursing. Cue-based feeds allow the infant to begin trials of oral intake when demonstrating cues. This may occur earlier than 34 weeks' gestation (58). Four major criteria determine readiness for oral feeding (59,60). (See Box 3.8.) Successful achievement in all four areas is important.

Box 3.8 Criteria to Determine Readiness for Nutritive Feeding

Age

- 32–34+ weeks' gestation: the typical age infants begin to demonstrate coordination of suck-swallow-breathe

Physiological

- Tolerates feeding into stomach
- Maintains consistent weight gain with tube feeding
- On ≤ 2 L oxygen due to concern that with increased flow, infants may be less able to protect their airway. If > 2 L, may be a candidate for introduction of tastes via pacifier dipped in human milk or formula
- Respiratory rate between 20–50 breaths per minute (bpm) but no more than 70 bpm; respiratory rate that is consistently more than 60 bpm may lead to reduced coordination of suck-swallow-breathe
- Stable work of breathing (no retractions, head bobbing, etc.)

State

- Ability to reach and maintain a quiet alert state

Maturational

- Tolerates handling and transitions without excessive signs of stress
- Root and nonnutritive suck emerging or established

Source: Used with permission. Data are from references 59 and 60.

Infants attempting oral feeds who are exhibiting behaviors or clinical signs that are concerning for aspiration or safety with feeding may need further evaluation. There are two common instrumental assessment tools to assess swallow function: the video swallow study (61,62) and the fiberoptic evaluation of swallow study (63,64). In addition, there is an informal tool to assess swallow function in patients with a tracheostomy that involves use of a dye test. However, this informal method has a high false-negative rate (65). See Box 3.9 (61,63).

Box 3.9 Assessments of Swallow Function

Video Swallow Study (VSS)
Description: Dynamic fluoroscopic images of 3 phases of swallowing (oral, pharyngeal, esophageal). Performed in radiology by radiologist and speech pathologist.
Advantages:

- No discomfort
- Observes each phase of swallow, coordination with respiration, and the impact of each aspect on the other
- Simulates a typical feeding
- Ability to trial compensatory strategies during the study (nipples, positioning, pacing, thickness of feeding)

Disadvantages:

- Exposure to radiation
- Unable to view swallowing of secretions
- Unrealistic for evaluation of infants whose intake is very limited

Appropriate populations: Infants who are able to take some volume of their feeding orally (formula/human milk)
Inappropriate populations: Infants who require evaluation of their secretion management

---

Fiberoptic Evaluation of Swallow Study (FEES)
Description: Transnasal passage of endoscope into hypopharynx, allowing assessment of the anatomy of pharynx, supraglottic larynx, and vocal cord function during swallow. Performed by otolaryngologist and speech pathologist.
Advantages:

- No radiation
- Observes anatomy and its function
- Observes infants' swallow function with management of secretions

(continued)

Box 3.9 Assessments of Swallow Function (continued)

Fiberoptic Evaluation of Swallow Study (FEES) (continued)
Disadvantages:

- Discomfort of passage/placement of endoscope
- Invasive
- Inability to evaluate oral or esophageal phases of swallow
- Possibility of scope affecting function
- Difficulty with observing sequential swallows in bottle feeding

Appropriate populations: Infants with swallow function concerns regarding secretion management and who are NPO
Inappropriate populations: Infants with nasal obstruction

Source: Data are from references 61 and 63.

Thickened Liquids

Despite many challenges and concerns with the use of thickened liquids, they are often used in the NICU. From a safety standpoint, premature infants have immunoreactive intestinal mucosa that place them at risk for infection and injury (66). The use of a popular xanthan gum–based thickening agent was recalled following concerns for NEC that resulted in 3 deaths in NICU infants (66).

From a clinical practice standpoint, thickened liquids are difficult to mix to a similar consistency with each presentation despite use of a recipe. Thickened liquids vary significantly (67–69) based on:

- Base liquid (human milk vs formula)
- Caloric density
- Product used to thicken (starch-based vs gum-based)
- Temperature of the liquid, and
- Setting time of the mixture

As a result, thickened liquids may vary from feeding to feeding. The infant must be able to adjust to the variability, accept the goal volume, and utilize it for growth. Additionally, the bottle and nipple system must allow the increased viscosity to flow easily. There are commercially available nipples that are "Y-cut," that are recommended for use with thickened feeds, such as those manufactured by Dr. Brown's (www.drbrownsbaby.com). Artificial enlargement of a nipple for feeding is not a safe practice. Best practice is to avoid use of thickened liquids unless specific circumstances prevent feeding without their use.

Late Preterm Infants

Late preterm infants (LPI) are defined as babies born between 34 0/7 and 36 6/7 weeks' gestation and are physiologically immature (70,71). Medical complications include, but are not limited to, respiratory distress, hyperbilirubinemia, hypoglycemia, and thermoregulation, all of which may impact the success of oral feeding and prolong hospitalization (72). Caregivers of LPIs require education regarding feeding readiness, coordination of sucking, swallowing and breathing, endurance, and state of arousal management. Families should demonstrate a clear understanding of the feeding plan (73). It is also recommended that LPIs consistently exhibit successful oral feeding prior to discharge (71). Nutrition is very important in LPIs as their brain size is 2/3 of the size of term infants (74). Nutritional recommendations are available and include 115 to 130 kcal/kg per day, 2.5 to 3.1 g protein/kg per day and 70 to 140 mg/kg calcium per day (75). Parent and professional education on this topic is available (76).

Nipples and Bottles

Nipples and bottles are considered based on their characteristics, matching the function to the individual infant. Nipples vary in shape, size, texture, and the type, size and number of holes. Once a bottle and nipple combination has been determined to be functional based on the individual infant's needs, it should be used consistently. To ensure consistency of flow, nipples should not be cut or otherwise altered. Prior to discharge, some babies may benefit from being transitioned to the bottle and nipple that will work best for them at home. Hospitals have policies in place to ensure proper sanitizing of these multiuse bottles and nipples, in contrast to the disposable products typically used in the hospital.

HYPERCALORIC FEEDINGS

Neonatal dietitians are challenged with providing optimal feedings to support proportional growth for infants who require fluid restriction or have nutrition needs more than what can be supplied with ready-to-feed formulas or concentrated liquids or powder products made according to manufacturers' directions. High-calorie feedings can be made by concentrating the formula and using less water, thereby keeping all nutrients in balance. High-calorie formulas can also be made using modular products, such as individual supplements of carbohydrate, protein, or fat, or a combination of carbohydrate and fat. Using modular supplements may alter the original balance of nutrients, but may be desired for clinical reasons. When altering formula concentration, it is very important to analyze nutrient composition to ensure desired nutrient intake, monitor tolerance and clinical status of the infant, and limit hang time to 4 hours (77). Box 3.2 has information about modular products.

Options for increasing the caloric density of human milk include:

- Use of commercially available HMF up to 24 kcal/oz (most common)
- Use of 30-calories-per-ounce preterm infant formula mixed with human milk or fortified human milk to make desired concentrations
- Use of hindmilk; estimate caloric density using the creamatocrit technique (78); special equipment is available but not required (The Creamatocrit Plus; Medela, Inc; www.separationtechnology.com/creamatocritplus.html)
- Use of powdered formula, concentrated liquid formula, or modular products that add carbohydrate, protein, and/or fat

Table 3.6 has several hypercaloric mixtures. These examples are for illustration purposes only. Consult manufacturers' websites, product handbooks, and product labels for possible changes in nutrient composition.

Table 3.6 Intake of Key Nutrients from Selected Hypercaloric Mixtures When Fed at 120 kcal/kg to a Hypothetical 1.5-kg Infant

Feeding	Volume mL/kg	Macronutrients g/kg	Micronutrients
24 kcal/oz Term HM with Similac HMF (Hydrolysate)[a]	150	CHO: 12.8 PRO: 3.8 Fat: 5.9	Na: 2 mEq/kg Ca: 185 mg/kg Fe: 0.6 mg/kg
26 kcal/oz Neocate[b]	138	CHO: 14 PRO: 3.7 Fat: 5.4	Na: 1.9 mEq/kg Ca: 149 mg/kg Fe: 2.2 mg/kg

(continued)

Table 3.6 Intake of Key Nutrients from Selected Hypercaloric Mixtures When Fed at 120 kcal/kg to a Hypothetical 1.5-kg Infant (continued)

24 kcal/oz Pregestimil + MCT Oil to make 28 kcal/oz[c]	129	CHO: 10.5 PRO: 2.9 Fat: 7.8	Na: 2.1 mEq/kg Ca: 97 mg/kg Fe: 1.9 mg/kg
20 kcal/oz Similac PM 60/40 + Duocal = 24 kcal/oz[d]	150	CHO: 13.2 PRO: 2.2 Fat: 6.5	Na: 1 mEq/kg Ca: 56 mg/kg Fe: 0.7 mg/kg
Term HM Mixed 1:1 with Similac Special Care 30[e]	142	CHO: 10.7 PRO: 2.9 Fat: 7.5	Na: 1.9 mEq/kg Ca: 149 mg/kg Fe: 1.3 mg/kg
20 cal/oz Good Start plus 2 tsp. Gerber Rice Cereal added /1 fl oz formula[f]	127	CHO 17.3 PRO: 2.4 Fat: 4.4	Na: 0.9 mEq/kg Ca: 107 mg/kg Fe: 5.2 mg/kg

Abbreviations: HM, human milk; HMF, human milk fortifier; CHO, carbohydrate; PRO, protein; Na, sodium; Ca, calcium; Fe, iron; MCT, medium-chain triglyceride

[a]Selected Indication: Added nutrient density for growing preterm infant up to term baby weight. Manufacturer: Abbott Nutrition

[b]Selected Indication: Concentrated elemental formula for allergy, short gut, or other gastro-intestinal problems. Manufacturer: Nutricia

[c]Selected Indication: Concentrated semielemental formula when additional MCT oil is needed in cases of liver failure, cholestasis, or chylothorax. Manufacturers. Mead Johnson and Nestle Nutrition

[d]Selected Indication: Low renal solute load formula with added nonprotein calories indicated in renal failure. Manufacturers: Abbott Nutrition and Nutricia

[e]Selected Indication: Fortified human milk made with hypercaloric premature formula to extend mother's milk; additional protein or micronutrients may be needed. Manufacturer: Abbott Nutrition

[f]Selected Indication: Thickened feeding used for reflux or swallowing problems but not recommended by this author; cereal textures and nutrient compositions vary. Formulas designed to assist with reflux are available and preferable over adding rice cereal (Enfamil AR, Similac Spit Up). Manufacturer: Gerber

Source: Data generated by WebNova, Abbott Nutrition, 2014. Nutrient values rounded to the nearest tenth.

Preparation of High-Calorie Feedings

Consider the following factors when preparing high-calorie feedings:

- Desired caloric density and desired final volume.
- Osmolality, especially with added medications. Monitor for possible adverse effects.
- Availability of equipment to measure ingredients precisely for hospitalized infants (gram scale for powders; mL precision for liquids).
- Concentrated liquid formulas are packaged in 13-fl oz cans (390 mL) and provide 1.33 kcal/mL (40 kcal/oz). Availability of concentrated liquid products are limited.
- Infant formula powders vary from 4.2 kcal/g to 5.2 kcal/g; when mixed with liquids, they range in volume displacement from 6.1 to 7.4 mL per scoop (for formulas prepared with 1 scoop per 2 oz water). Measuring instructions may indicate packed or unpacked powder (79).
- Conversion to recipes using scoops and household measurements for preparation at home.

Safety Issues

Consider the following safety issues when preparing all infant feedings:

- Powdered formulas and human milk fortifiers are not commercially sterile and should not be used in the NICU setting or in infants who are immunocompromised unless there is no nutritionally appropriate alternative available. If fortification of human milk or a formula must be made using a powder, care must be taken to minimize the risk of bacterial contamination and proliferation (80). To do so, mix the smallest volume possible—one feeding at a time is preferred—and minimize the holding time (at room temperature or refrigerated). Use the smallest amount of powder possible. For example, if mixing NeoSure 24 kcal/oz, add the correct amount of NeoSure powder to NeoSure 22 ready-to-feed to achieve 24 kcal/oz, rather than mixing NeoSure powder with sterile water to make 24 kcal/oz.

- Manufacturers have specific recommendations related to the handling of their products as well as the recommended amount of time their products should be kept at room temperature once reconstituted. Guidelines have been developed to promote the safest feeding preparation and storage practices (60,77).
- When available, a sterile ready-to-feed or concentrated liquid formula or human milk fortifier is recommended for use with all infants. (See Box 3.3 and Table 3.1.)
- Formulas made in the hospital should be stored in food-grade materials, such as glass, plastic, or milk cartons. A variety of suitable bottles and lids are available from dairies, formula manufacturers, and container companies. See the Human Milk Storage section earlier in this chapter.

POTENTIAL RENAL SOLUTE LOAD AND OSMOLALITY

Potential renal solute load (PRSL) is the amount of nitrogen from protein plus the sum of sodium, potassium, chloride, and phosphorus that a feeding contains. PRSL is expressed as mOsm/L or mOsm/100 kcal (81). Equations to calculate PRSL are available (82). Actual renal solute load can be calculated, assuming not all renal solute load (RSL) is presented to the kidney when the infant is growing. Urine osmolality can be estimated from actual RSL (82). Feedings with a high PRSL could increase the risk of dehydration. The upper limit of PRSL for infant feedings is 277 mOsm/L or 30 to 35 mOsm/100 kcal (82–84).

Osmolality is a measurement of the concentration of solutes in solution. Values are expressed as mOsm/kg water. The osmolality of blood is about 300 mOsm/kg water. Hyperosmolar feedings may cause intolerance and diarrhea. Carbohydrate as monosaccharides and disaccharides are major contributors to osmolality.

Medications and vitamin/mineral supplements in syrups are extremely hyperosmolar (85). The final osmolality of formula-medication mixtures can be calculated (86). To reduce the osmolality of feedings with added syrup-based medications, divide the medication dose or use another form of the medication, such as IV. Be aware that an electronic medical record system may default to adding all supplements and medications to one feeding, which could potentially result in a dangerously high osmolality. The upper limit of osmolality suggested, but not universally supported, for infant feedings is 450 mOsm/kg water (as estimated from an osmolarity of 400 mOsm/L) (1,87).

SUMMARY

- Human milk is the preferred feeding for all newborns. Human milk fed to infants who are ≤ 34 weeks' gestational age or weigh ≤ 1,500 g at birth should be fortified with a commercial human milk fortifier.
- Commercial infant formulas are used if human milk is not available. Preterm infants are fed with pre-

term infant formulas unless those products are not tolerated.

- Vitamin/mineral supplements may be indicated in selected situations and are most commonly fat-soluble vitamins, especially vitamin D, and the minerals calcium, phosphorus, iron, and zinc.
- Enteral feedings are delivered to preterm infants by gavage with transition to breast or bottle at approximately 34 to 36 weeks' gestational age.
- Noncommercial enteral feedings must be carefully designed for nutritional adequacy, prepared using strictly controlled policies and procedures, and delivered in a timely fashion to ensure safety and efficacy.

REFERENCES

1. American Academy of Pediatrics Committee on Nutrition. In: Kleinman RE, Greer FR, eds. *Pediatric Nutrition*. 7th ed. Elk Grove Village, IL: American Academy of Pediatrics; 2014.
2. Tudehope DI. Human milk and the nutritional needs of preterm infants. *J Pediatr*. 2013; 162;3(Suppl 1):S17–S25
3. The Academy of Breastfeeding Medicine Board of Directors. Position on Breastfeeding. *Breastfeeding Medicine*. 2008;3(4):267–270.
4. Sisk PM, Lovelady CA, Dillard RG, Gruber KJ, O'Shea TM. Early human milk feeding is associated with a lower risk of necrotizing enterocolitis in very low birth weight infants. *J Perinatol.* 2007;27:428–433.
5. Meinzen-Derr J, Poindexter B, Wrage L, Morrow AL, Stoll B, Donovan EF. Role of human milk in extremely low birth weight infants' risk of necrotizing enterocolitis or death. *J Perinatol.* 2009;29:57–62.
6. Hylander MA, Strobino DM, Dhanireddy R. Human milk feedings and infection among very low birth weight infants. *Pediatrics*. 1998;102:e38.
7. Lawrence RA, Lawrence RM, eds. *Breastfeeding: A Guide for the Medical Profession.* 7th ed. St. Louis, MO: Mosby; 2011.

8. Lawrence RM, Lawrence RA. Breastfeeding: More Than Just Good Nutrition. *Pediatr Rev.* 2011;32(7):267–279
9. American Academy of Pediatrics. Health Initiatives. *Breastfeeding: Policy on Breastfeeding and Use of Human Milk.* www.aap.org. Accessed March 24, 2015.
10. Cincinnati Children's Center for Breastfeeding Medicine. www.cincinnatichildrens.org/service/c/breastfeeding/services/. Accessed March 24 2015.
11. Lessen R, Sapsford A. Expressed human milk. In Robins S, Meyers R, eds. *Infant Feedings: Guidelines for Preparation of Human Milk and Formula in Health Care Facilities*. Chicago, IL: American Dietetic Association; 2011:40–70.
12. Human Milk Banking Association of North America. *2011 Best Practice for Expressing, Storing and Handling Human Milk in Hospitals, Homes, and Child Care Settings*. www.hmbana.org /publications. Accessed March 24, 2015.
13. National Biomonitoring Program, Bisphenol A Fact Sheet. Centers for Disease Control and Prevention. www.cdc.gov/bio monitoring/BisphenolA_FactSheet.html. Accessed March 24, 2015.
14. Slutzah M, Codipilly CN, Potak D, Clark RM, Schanler JJ. Refrigerator storage of expressed human milk in the neonatal intensive care unit. *J Pediatr*. 2010;156(1):26–28.
15. Centers for Disease Control and Prevention. Breastfeeding Proper Handling and Storage of Human Milk. www.cdc.gov /breastfeeding/recommendations/handling_breastmilk.htm. Accessed March 19, 2015.
16. United States Department of Agriculture, Food Safety and Inspection Service. Food Safety Information. Refrigeration and Food Safety. www.fsis.usda.gov/wps/wcm/connect/934c2c81–2a3d –4d59–b6ce–c238fdd45582/Refrigeration_and_Food_Safety .pdf?MOD=AJPERES. Accessed March 24, 2015.
17. Penguin. http://crecheinnovations.com/products/overview. Accessed March 24, 2015.
18. Waterless Milk Warmer. www.medelabreastfeedingus.com /for-professionals/products/516/waterless-milk-warmer. Accessed March 24, 2015.
19. Dumm M, Hamms M, Sutton J, Ryan-Wenger N. NICU breast milk warming practices and the physiological effects of breast milk feeding temperatures on preterm infants. *Adv Neonatal Care*. 2013;13:279–287.

20. 2015 Hospital 5 National Patient Safety Goals. The Joint Commission. www.jointcommission.org/hap_2015_npsgs. Accessed March 24, 2015.
21. Groh-Wargo S, Sapsford A. Enteral nutritional support of the preterm infant in the neonatal intensive care unit. *Nutr Clin Pract*. 2009;24:363–376.
22. Valentine CJ, Morrow G, Pennel M, Morrow AL, Hodge A, Haban-Bartz A, Collins K, Rogers LK. Randomized controlled trial of docosahexaenoic acid supplementation in Midwestern U.S. milk donors. *Breastfeed Med*. 2013;8(1):86–91.
23. Fusch G, Rochow N, Choi A, Fusch S, Poeschl S, Ubah A, Lee S, Raja P, Fusch C. Rapid measurement of macronutrients in breast milk: How reliable are infrared milk analyzers? *Clinical Nutrition*. 2014;5:465–476. http://dx.doi.org/10.1016/j.clnu.2014.05.005.
24. Schanler, RJ, Lau C, Hurst NM, Smith EO. Randomized trial of donor human milk versus preterm formula as substitutes for mothers' own milk in the feeding of extremely premature infants. *Pediatrics*. 2005;116:400–406.
25. Cincinnati Children's Hospital Medical Center. Evidence-based care guideline for necrotizing enterocolitis (NEC) among very low birth weight infants. Cincinnati (OH): Cincinnati Children's Hospital Medical Center; 2010. www.guideline.gov/content.aspx?id=24815&search=nec+cincinnati. Accessed March 24, 2015.
26. Lucas A, Cole TJ. Breastmilk and neonatal necrotizing enterocolitis. *Lancet*. 1990;336:1519–1523.
27. Quigley M, Henderson G, Anthony M, McGuire W. Formula milk versus donor breast milk for feeding preterm or low birth weight infants. *Cochrane Database Syst Rev*. 2007;(4):CD002971
28. Human Milk Banking Association of North America. www.hmbana.org. Accessed March 24, 2015.
29. Geraghty SR, McNamara KA, Dillon CE, Hogan JS, Kwiek JJ, Keim SA. Buying human milk via the internet: just a click away. *Breastfeed Med*. 2013;8:1–5.
30. Sullivan S, Schanler RJ, Kim JH, Patel AL, Trawöger R, Kiechl-Kohlendorfer U, Chan GM, Blanco CL, Abrams S, Cotten CM, Laroia N, Ehrenkranz RA, Dudell G, Cristofalo EA, Meier P, Lee ML, Rechtman DJ, Lucas A. An exclusively human milk-based diet is associated with a lower rate of necrotizing enterocolitis

than a diet of human milk and bovine milk-based products. *J Pediatr*. 2010;156:562–567.

31. Tudehope D, Fewtrell M, Kashyap S, Udaeta E. Nutritional needs of the micropreterm infant. *J Peds*. 2013;162(Suppl 3):S72–S80.
32. Brown LD, Hendrickson K, Masor ML, Hay WW. High–protein formulas: Evidence for use in preterm infants. *Clin Perinatol*. 2014;41:383–403.
33. Bhatia J, Greer F, and the Committee on Nutrition. Use of soy protein-based formulas in infant feeding. *Pediatrics*. 2008;121:1062–1068.
34. Mihatsch WA, Franz AR, Hogel J, Pohlandt F. Hydrolyzed protein accelerates feeding advancement in very low birth weight infants. *Pediatrics*. 2002;110:1199–1203.
35. Joeckel RK, Phillips SK. Overview of infant and pediatric formulas. *Nutr in Clin Pract*. 2009;24(3): 356–362
36. Wright B, Begany M, Kinne J. Selected children's multivitamin and mineral supplements. *ICAN: Infant, Child & Adolescent Nutrition*. 2011;3(2):102–115.
37. Merhar LS, Meinzen-Derr J, Sprague J, Wessel JJ, Leugers S, Painter J, Valentine CJ. Safety and tolerability of enteral protein supplementation for infants with brain injury. *Nutr Clin Prac*. 2015; PMID 25616519. Accessed May 5, 2015.
38. Tsang RC, Uauy R, Koletzko B, Zlotkin SH. *Nutrition of the Preterm Infant: Scientific Basis and Practical Guidelines*. 2nd ed. Cincinnati, OH: Digital Educational Publishing; 2005.
39. Koletzko B, Poindexter B, Uauy R, eds. In: Koletzko B, ed. *Nutritional Care of Preterm Infants: Scientific Basis and Practical Guidelines*. Basel, Switzerland: Karger; 2014. *World Review of Nutrition and Dietetics*. vol 110.
40. Agostoni C, Buonocore G, Carnielli VP, De Curtis M, Darmaun D, Decsi T, Domellöf M, Embleton ND, Fusch C, Genzel-Boroviczeny O, Goulet O, Kalhan SC, Kolacek S, Koletzko B, Lapillonne A, Mihatsch W, Moreno L, Neu J, Poindexter B, Puntis J, Putet G, Rigo J, Riskin A, Salle B, Sauer P, Shamir R, Szajewska H, Thureen P, Turck D, van Goudoever JB, Ziegler EE; for ESPGHAN Committee on Nutrition. Enteral nutrient supply for preterm infants: commentary from the European Society for Paediatric Gastroenterology, Hepatology, and Nutrition Committee on Nutrition. *J Pediatr Gastroenterol Nutr*. 2010;50(1):85–91.

41. Institute of Medicine. Dietary Reference Intakes: Summary Tables. http://iom.edu/Activities/Nutrition/SummaryDRIs/~/media/Files/Activity%20Files/Nutrition/DRIs/New%20Material/5DRI%20Values%20SummaryTables%2014.pdf Accessed March 24, 2015.
42. Misra M, Pacaud D, Petryk A, Collett-Solberg PF, Kappy M. Drug and Therapeutics Committee of the Lawson Wilkins Pediatric Endocrine Society. Vitamin D deficiency in children and its management: review of current knowledge and recommendations. *Pediatrics*. 2008;122(2):398–417.
43. Golden N, Abrams S, Committee on Nutrition. Optimizing bone health in children and adolescents. *Pediatrics*. 2014;134(4):e1229–e1243. doi: 10.1542/peds.2014–2173.
44. Food and Drug Administration. *Public Health Notification: PVC devices containing the plasticizer DEHP*. July 2002. www.fda.gov/MedicalDevices/Safety/AlertsandNotices/PublicHealthNotifications/ucm062182.htm. Accessed March 24, 2015.
45. Parker P, Stroop S, Greene H. A controlled comparison of continuous versus intermittent feeding in the treatment of infants with intestinal disease. *J Pediatr.* 1987;99:360–365.
46. Heyman MB, Harmatz P, Acree M, Wilson L, Moskowitz JT, Ferrando S, Folkman S. Economic and psychologic costs for maternal caregivers of gastrostomy–dependent children. *J Pediatr.* 2004;145:511–516.
47. Maggio L, Costa S, Zecca C, Giordano L. Methods of Enteral Feeding in Preterm Infants. *Early Hum Dev*. 2012;88(Suppl 2):S31–33.
48. Rogers SP, Hicks PD, Hamzo M, Veit LE, Abrams SA. Continuous Feedings of Fortified Human Milk Lead to Nutrient Losses of Fat, Calcium and Phosphorus. *Nutrients*. 2010;2:230–240.
49. The Joint Commission. *Managing Risk During Transition to New ISO Tubing Connector Standards*. Sentinel Event Alert Issue 53. August 20, 2014. www.jointcommission.org/sea_issue_53/. Accessed March 24, 2015.
50. Ryan CA, Mohammad I, Murphy B. Normal neurologic and developmental outcome after accidental intravenous infusion of expressed breast milk in a neonate. *Pediatrics.* 2006;117:236–238.
51. Guenter P. New Enteral Connectors: Raising Awareness. *Nutr Clin Pract.* 2014;29(5):612–614.

52. Boullata J, Carney LN, Guenter P, eds. *A.S.P.E.N. Enteral Nutrition Handbook.* Silver Spring, MD: American Society for Parenteral and Enteral Nutrition; 2010.
53. Copelan D, Appel J. Implementation of an enteral nutrition and medication administration system utilizing oral syringes in the NICU. *Neonatal Netw.* 2006;25:21–25.
54. Berseth CL, Bisquera JA, Paje VU. Prolonging small feeding volumes early in life decreases the incidence of necrotizing enterocolitis in very low birth weight infants. *Pediatrics.* 2003;111:529–534.
55. Meetze WH, Valentine C, McGuigan JE, Conlon M, Sacks N, Neu J. Gastrointestinal priming prior to full enteral nutrition in very low birth weight infants. *J Pediatr Gastroenterol Nutr.* 1992;15:163–170.
56. Torrazza RM, Parker LA, Li Y, Talaga E, Shuster J, Neu J. The value of routine evaluation of gastric residuals in very low birth weight infants. *J Perinatol.* 2014;1–4.
57. Hanson C, Sundermeier J, Dugick L, Lyden E, Anderson-Berry AL. Implementation, process, and outcomes of nutrition best practices for infants <1500g. *Nutr Clin Pract.* 2011;26:614–624.
58. Ludwig SM, Waitzman KA. Changing feeding documentation to reflect infant-driven feeding practice. *Newborn and Infant Nursing Reviews*. 2007;7(3):155–160.
59. Shaker CS, Werner Woida AM. An evidence–based approach to nipple feeding in a level III NICU: nurse autonomy, developmental care, and teamwork. *Neonatal Netw.* 2001;26:77–83.
60. Lemons PK. From gavage to oral feedings: just a matter of time. *Neonatal Netw.* 2001;3:7–14.
61. Arvedson JC, Lefton-Greif M. *Pediatric Videofluoroscopic Swallow Studies: A Professional Manual with Caregiver Guidelines.* San Antonio, TX: Communication Skill Builders; 1998.
62. Logemann J. *Evaluation and Treatment of Swallowing Disorders.* Austin, TX: Pro-Ed, 1998.
63. Leder S, Karas D. Fiberoptic endoscopic evaluation of swallowing in the pediatric population. *Larygoscope.* 2000;110: 1132–1136.
64. Hartnick K, Kartley B, Miller C, Willging JP. Pediatric fiberoptic endoscopic evaluation of swallowing. *Ann Otol Rhinol Laryngol.* 2000;109:996–999.

65. O'Neil-Pirozzi TM, Lisiecki DJ, Momose KJ, Connors JJ, Milliner MP. Simultaneous modified barium swallow and blue dye tests: a determination of the accuracy of blue dye test aspiration findings. *Dysphagia.* 2003;18:32–38.
66. Woods CW, Oliver T, Lewis K, Yang Q. Development of necrotizing enterocolitis in premature infants receiving thickened feeds using SimplyThick®. *J Perinatol.* 2012;32:150–152.
67. Cichero JAY, Nicholson TM, September C. Thickened milk for the management of feeding and swallowing issues in infants: a call for interdisciplinary professional guidelines. *J Hum Lact.* 2013;29(2):132–135.
68. Garcia JM, Chambers E, Matta Z, Clark M. Serving temperature viscosity measurements of nectar- and honey-thick liquids. *Dysphagia.* 2008;23:65–75.
69. Stuart S, Motz JM. Viscosity of infant dysphagia management: comparison of viscosity of thickened liquids used in assessment and thickened liquids used in treatment. *Dysphagia* 2009;24:412–422.
70. Engle WA. A recommendation for the definition of "late preterm" (near-term) and the birth weight-gestational age classification system. *Semin Perinatol.* 2006;30(1):2–7.
71. Engle WA, Tomashek KM, Wallman C. "Late-preterm" infants: a population at risk. *Pediatrics.* 2007;120:1390–1401.
72. Cleaveland K. Feeding Challenges in the late preterm infant. *Neonatal Netw.* 2010;29(1):37–41.
73. Raju TNK, Higgins RD, Stark AR, Leveno KJ. Optimizing care and outcome for late-preterm (near-term) infants: a summary of the workshop sponsored by the National Institute of Child Health and Human Development. *Pediatrics.* 2006;118:1207–1214.
74. Loftin RW, Habli M, Snyder CC, Cormier CM, Lewis DF, DeFranco EA. Late preterm birth. *Rev Obstet Gynecol.* 2010;3(1):10–19.
75. Lapillonne A, O'Connor DL, Wang D, Rigo J. Nutritional recommendations for the late pre-term infant and the preterm infant after discharge. *J Pediatr.* 2013;162:S90–100.
76. March of Dimes. www.marchofdimes.org/catalog/product.aspx?productcode=37-2229-07. Accessed March 24, 2015.
77. Hutsler D, Benson-Szekely L. Delivery and bedside management of infant feedings. In Robbins ST, Meyers R, eds. *Infant*

Feedings: Guidelines for Preparation of Human Milk and Formula in Health Care Facilities. 2nd ed. Chicago: American Dietetic Association, Pediatric Nutrition Practice Group; 2011:95–107.

78. Meier PP, Engstrom JL, Murtaugh MA, Vasan U, Meier WA, Schanler RJ. Mothers' milk feedings in the neonatal intensive care unit: accuracy of the creamatocrit technique. *J Perinatol.* 2002;22:646–649.
79. Academy of Nutrition and Dietetics. Pediatric Nutrition Care Manual. Formulary, Formula Mixing Recipes. https://www.nutritioncaremanual.org/vault/2440/web/files/CCHMC%20Formula%20Charts%20August%202014.pdf. Accessed March 26, 2015.
80. Food and Drug Administration. *Health Professionals Letter on* Enterobacter sakazakii *Infections Associated with Use of Powdered (Dry) Infant Formulas in Neonatal Intensive Care Units.* April/October 2002. www.fda.gov/Food/RecallsOutbreaks Emergencies/SafetyAlertsAdvisories/ucm111299.htm. Accessed March 24, 2015.
81. Fomon SJ. Potential renal solute load: considerations relating to complementary feedings of breastfed infants. *Pediatrics.* 2000;106:1284.
82. Fomon JS, Ziegler EE. Water and renal solute load. In: Fomon SJ, ed. *Nutrition of Normal Infants.* St Louis, MO: Mosby; 1993:91–102.
83. Fomon SJ, Ziegler EE. Renal solute load and potential renal solute load in infancy. *J Pediatr.* 1999;134:11–14.
84. Assessment of nutrient requirements for infant formulas (erratum in: *J Nutr.* 1999;129:1090). *J Nutr.* 1998;128(Suppl 11):S2059–S2293.
85. Radmacher PG, Adamkin MD, Lewis ST, Adamkin DH. Milk as a vehicle for oral medications: hidden osmoles. *J Perinatol.* 2012;32:227–239.
86. Jew RK, Owen D, Kaufman D, Balmer D. Osmolality of commonly used medications and formulas in the neonatal intensive care unit. *Nutr Clin Pract.* 1997;12:158–163.
87. Pearson F, Johnson MJ, Leaf AA. Milk osmolality: does it matter? *Arch Dis Child Fetal Neonatal Ed.* 2013;98(2):F166–169.

Chapter 4

Medical/Surgical Conditions Introduction

Janice Hovasi Cox, MS, RD, CSP

OBJECTIVES

- Describe nutrition related strategies that help prevent medical complications common in high-risk newborns and/or preterm infants.
- Describe nutrition related strategies to treat congenital anomalies, disease states, and/or surgical interventions in high-risk newborns and/or preterm infants.

INTRODUCTION

Each of the following 12 chapters has a similar format, as follows:

- Brief description of the disease state or condition and its nutrition implications
- Preventive nutrition
- Treatment nutrition

Although this is the general format, individual sections may have slight variations as appropriate to their content.

These chapters use the simplified evidence-based medicine rating system called the Strength of Recommendation Taxonomy (SORT). The ABC rating scale of the SORT is applicable to neonatal intensive care unit (NICU) nutrition content, easy to use and remember, and well documented. The rating scale, described in more detail elsewhere (1–3), includes:

- Level **A** (randomized, controlled trials; meta-analyses)
- Level **B** (other evidence, such as high-quality non-randomized trials, cohort studies, case-control studies, and retrospective studies)
- Level **C** (consensus viewpoint, expert opinion, and usual practice)

The evidence levels have been assigned by the chapter authors and are included as **(A)**, **(B)**, or **(C)** following recommendations in this chapter.

REFERENCES

1. Ebell MH, Siwek J, Weiss BD, Woolf SH, Susman J, Ewigman B, Bowman M. Strength of Recommendation Taxonomy (SORT): a patient-centered approach to grading evidence in the medical literature. *J Am Board Fam Pract.* 2004;17:59–67.
2. SORT: The strength-of-recommendation taxonomy. *Am Fam Physician.* 2006;74:17–18.
3. Ebell MH, Siwek J, Weiss BD, Woolf SH, Susman JL, Ewigman B, Bowman M. Simplifying the language of evidence to improve patient care. *J Fam Pract.* 2004;53:111–120.

Chapter 5

Respiratory Disease

Janice Hovasi Cox, MS, RD, CSP

DISEASE STATE

Respiratory distress syndrome (RDS) is characterized by cyanosis in room air, nasal flaring, grunting, retracting, and tachypnea. RDS may develop in preterm infants due to immaturity of lung tissue structure and function. Alveoli surface area is smaller not only due to size, but also due to a relative lack of alveolar surfactant. Surfactant allows improved expansion of alveoli during inspiration. Supplemental oxygen or pressure used to treat respiratory compromise can also cause inflammation and tissue damage (1,2). Other causes of RDS during the newborn period are meconium aspiration, pneumonia, lung hypoplasia, transient tachypnea, pneumothorax, or chylous pleural effusion (1).

RDS may progress to bronchopulmonary dysplasia (BPD), sometimes called chronic lung disease of prematurity (CLD). BPD may be defined by supplemental oxygen > 21% dependency for ≥ 28 days or beyond 36 weeks' gestational age (GA) for infants < 32 weeks' GA at birth. It may be mild, moderate, or severe depending on the amount of oxygen support required and presence of other lung function abnormalities. Infants born between 23 and 30 weeks' GA are at greatest risk for BPD because oxygen and pressure delivery, infection, fluids, and nutrient deficits may interfere with normal lung development, resulting in fewer, though larger, alveoli, and a smaller gas exchange surface area. Although lung tissue continues to grow and remodel, resulting in gradual improvement, symptoms may continue into adolescence (2–4). Preterm infants with intrauterine growth restriction (IUGR) may be more likely to develop both RDS and BPD. Depending on the duration and severity of impaired fetal oxygenation and nutrition, IUGR infants may have reduced levels of surfactant and decreased alveolar cell formation, maturation, and oxygen exchange surface area (5).

Infants with respiratory disease may have difficulty achieving adequate oral intake due to increased respiratory rate; difficulty coordinating an efficient and sustained suck, swallow, and breathing pattern; or early fatigue with feedings. Infants requiring mechanical ventilation or constant positive airway pressure ventilation (CPAP) for prolonged periods of time may develop feeding aversion, refuse oral feedings, or have difficulty with gag reflex or accepting foods with different textures.

Infants with BPD may have associated gastroesophageal reflux disease (GERD), which may result in microaspiration, esophagitis, or episodic bronchospasm—each of which may contribute to feeding aversion (1–6).

PREVENTIVE NUTRITION

Energy and Protein

Inadequate nutrient intake in very low birth weight (VLBW) infants decreases nutrient reserves and may adversely affect surfactant production; respiratory muscle function; and lung tissue growth, maturation, and repair. Meeting energy and protein needs promptly after birth may mediate the occurrence and severity of disease (7). For VLBW infants, provide 2.5 to 3.5 g protein/kg/day during the first 24 to 48 hours of life and 3.5 to 4 g/kg/day subsequently to support growth (8).

Fluids and Electrolytes

To help prevent pulmonary edema in preterm infants, allow initial diuresis to occur as evidenced by a 2.4% to 4% daily weight loss, up to a total weight loss 8% to 15% from initial weight during the first few days of life. Allowing diuresis generally requires limiting fluids initially to 70 to 80 mL/kg/d and adjusting daily, based on individual needs **(C)** (1,9). Late preterm and term infants with transient tachypnea also require initial fluid restrictions of 60 and 40 mL/kg/d, respectively. Adjust fluids as needed to prevent dehydration and hypovolemia. Increase fluids by 20 mL/kg/d until adequate feeding volumes are achieved **(C)** (10).

For preterm infants, restrict sodium to 0 to 1 mEq/kg/d during the first few days of life. Provide 1 to 2 mEq/kg/d after the onset of diuresis, and then increase as needed to maintain fluid and electrolyte balance **(A)** (1,6).

Vitamin A

Low serum and tissue vitamin A levels and low serum retinol binding protein levels in extremely low birth weight (ELBW) infants are associated with decreased clearance of lung secretions, abnormal tracheobronchial epithelium water homeostasis, loss of cilia, decreased ability to repair lung tissue injury, and increased incidence of BPD.

For ELBW infants, intramuscular (IM) administration of vitamin A—5,000 IU three times per week for 4 weeks for a total of 12 doses—may provide a modest reduction in the incidence of BPD **(A)** (11). Vitamin A has not been available as an IM preparation in recent years. Although it is currently available, acceptability of IM injections in ELBW infants and cost must be weighed against the modest benefit of this therapy (11).

Vitamin E

Research shows no benefit for supplementing intake of vitamin E beyond sustaining normal serum levels. Pharmacologic doses may be associated with increased risk of sepsis and necrotizing enterocolitis (NEC) **(B)** (12).

Inositol

Inositol plays a role in surfactant synthesis and epithelial cell growth, and may play a role as an antioxidant, although studies do not show respiratory benefit from supplementation (13).

Lipids

Protecting parenteral lipid infusion from light exposure or coadministration of parenteral lipids with multivitamin preparations may protect lung tissue and decrease chronic lung changes by limiting peroxide exposure, which may overload the capacity of the antioxidants that are present **(B)** (14).

TREATMENT NUTRITION

Energy

Initial intake should be 40 to 60 kcal/kg/d. Increase by day 6 to levels that support tissue accretion: 85 to 115 kcal/kg/d parenterally or 90 to 130 kcal/kg/d enterally **(C)** (8).

Subsequent intakes of 100 to 120 kcal/kg/d parenterally or 120 to 150 kcal/kg/d enterally may be needed to accommodate increased metabolic rate caused by the work of breathing and stress associated with compromised lung function **(B)** (8). Energy intakes > 125 to 135 kcal/kg/d or parenteral glucose infusions > 12 mg/kg/minute may increase work of breathing due to increased CO_2 production, and may not provide further benefit **(C)** (6,8,15,16).

Protein

In preterm infants, protein intake of at least 3.3 g/kg/d during the first 20 days of life may prevent early protein deficit, although intakes of 3.5 to 4 g/kg/d may be needed to support normal growth, including lean tissue accretion and organ growth **(C)** (17). These protein intakes positively affect protein balance, as evidenced by improved linear growth, but there is still a need for a more precise determination of lean tissue accretion and organ growth so that optimal protein requirements can be determined (18). Protein needs may be further increased during stress or steroid use **(C)** (19). For term infants with severe respiratory distress due to meconium aspiration or persistent pulmonary hypertension who require extracorporeal membrane oxygenation (ECMO), provide protein intake of 3 g/kg/d and at least 80 but not more than 100 kcal/kg/d **(B)** (20).

Lipids

Lipids may improve fat-soluble vitamin bioavailability and decrease carbon dioxide production by limiting conversion of carbohydrate to fat **(C)**.

Infants with chylothorax may require enteral feedings that limit or omit long-chain fatty acids. (See Chapter 6, Congenital Heart Disease, for additional information.)

If parenteral lipid emulsion is needed for infants receiving ECMO, provide through separate venous access to prevent agglutination and clot development within the ECMO circuit **(C)** (21).

Fluid Restriction

Beyond the initial 7 to 10 days of life, fluid tolerance may range from 120 to 150 mL/kg/d to prevent fluid retention, patency of the ductus arteriosus, pulmonary edema, and congestive heart failure **(A)** (6).

Increase nutrient density of formula or human milk to meet nutritional needs within tolerated feeding volume **(C)**. To achieve adequate nutrient intake, 24- to 30-kcal/oz concentrations of appropriate infant formula are recommended **(B)** (6,22,23). Supplementation with carbohydrate or fat additives to achieve adequate energy intake may decrease intake of other nutrients, particularly protein (6,22,23).

Human milk fortifiers, liquid protein fortifiers, and concentrated liquid formulas may be used as needed to increase nutrient density of human milk and maintain adequate nutrition when fluid restriction is needed **(C)**.

Feeding Problems

Enlist the support of a feeding therapist, who can provide care plans that reduce noxious oral-facial stimulation and recommend ways to enhance oral-motor development **(C)** (24).

Many infants with compromised respiratory function require prolonged use of enteral nutrition. Encourage flexible schedules for feedings to accommodate hunger and satiety cues **(C)**.

For postdischarge tube feedings, provide family and physician with expected weight gain and feeding guidelines to accommodate growth but prevent overfeeding **(C)**.

Drug-Nutrient Interactions

Drugs commonly used in the treatment of neonatal respiratory diseases include corticosteroids, diuretics, bronchodilators, and potassium replacement:

- Infants who demonstrate growth delay due to postnatal corticosteroid administration, specifically dexamethasone given systemically, may experience better growth recovery of lean tissue with higher protein intake **(C)**. Use of corticosteroids may cause hyperglycemia. If the patient receives parenteral nutrition, monitor serum glucose levels and modify glucose infusion and/or provide insulin as needed to maintain euglycemia.
- Use of chlorothiazide diuretics may cause delayed growth due to decreased serum levels of sodium, potassium, and chloride, requiring supplementation of these electrolytes. Use of spironolactone may elevate serum potassium, but may increase urinary sodium and chloride excretion. All diuretics increase renal phosphorus excretion, causing negative phosphorus balance and increasing the risk for osteopenia (25). Provide adequate phosphorus with the appropriate calcium to phosphorus ratio **(C)**. (See Chapter 15, Osteopenia of Prematurity, for further information.) When providing calcium supplements to infants receiving diuretics, use caution as this may cause nephrocalcinosis. Potassium supplements may be irritating to the gastrointestinal tract, causing vomiting, diarrhea, and bleeding.

REFERENCES

1. Sweet D, Bevilacqua G, Carnielli V, Greisen G, Plavka R, Didrik Saugstad O, Simeoni U, Speer CP, Valls-I-Soler A, Halliday H; Working Group on Prematurity of the World Association of Perinatal Medicine, European Association of Perinatal Medicine. European consensus guidelines on the management of neonatal respiratory distress syndrome. *J Perinat Med.* 2007;35:175–186.

2. Cox J. Nutrition in neonatal pulmonary disease. In: Dumont RC and Chung Y, eds. *Nutrition in pediatric pulmonary disease.* New York: Springer Science+Business Media. 2014;55–80.
3. Baraldi E, Filippone M. Chronic lung disease after premature birth. *N Engl J Med.* 2007;357:1946–1955.
4. Kair LR, Leonard DT, and Anderson JM. Bronchopulmonary dysplasia. *Pediatr Rev.* 2012;33:255–263.
5. Pike K, Pillow JJ, Lucas JS. Long term respiratory consequences of intrauterine growth restriction. *Semin Fetal Neonatal Med.* 2012;17:92–98.
6. Biniwale MA, Ehrenkranz RA. The role of nutrition in the prevention and management of bronchopulmonary dysplasia. *Semin Perinatol.* 2006;30:200–208.
7. Ehrenkranz RA, Das A, Wrage LA, Poindexter BB, Higgins RD, Stoll BJ, Oh W; Eunice Kennedy Shriver National Institute of Child Health and Human Development Neonatal Research Network. Early nutrition mediates the influence of severity of illness on extremely LBW infants. *Pediatr Res.* 2011:69:522–529.
8. Embleton ND. Optimal protein and energy intakes in preterm infants. *Early Hum Dev.* 2007;83;831–837.
9. Oh W. Fluid and electrolyte management of very low birth weight infants. *Pediatr Neonatol.* 2012;53(6):329–333
10. Stroustrup A, Trasande L, Holzman IR. Randomized controlled trial of restrictive fluid management in transient tachypnea of the newborn. *J Pediatr.* 2012;160:38–43.
11. Darlow BA, Graham PJ. Vitamin A supplementation to prevent mortality and short- and long-term morbidity in very low birthweight infants. *Cochrane Database Syst Rev.* 2011;(10):CD000501.
12. Brion LP, Bell EF, Raghuveer TS. Vitamin E supplementation for prevention of morbidity and mortality in preterm infants. *Cochrane Database Syst Rev.* 2003;4:CD003665.
13. Howlett A, Ohlsson A, Plakkal N. Inositol for respiratory distress syndrome in preterm infants. *Cochrane Database Syst Rev.* 2012;(3):CD000366.
14. Bassiouny MR, Almarsafawy H, Abdel-Hady H, Nasef N, Hammad TA, Aly H. A randomized controlled trial on parenteral nutrition, oxidative stress and chronic lung diseases in preterm infants. *J Pediatr Gastroenterol Nutr.* 2009;48:363–369.
15. Lai NM, Rajadurai SV, Tan KH. Increased energy intake for preterm infants with (or developing) bronchopulmonary

dysplasia/chronic lung disease. *Cochrane Database Syst Rev.* 2006;(3):CD005093.

16. Bhandari A, Bhandari V. Pitfalls, problems, and progress in bronchopulmonary dysplasia. *Pediatrics.* 2009;123:1562–1573.
17. Theile AR, Radmacher PG, Anschutz TW, Davis DW, Adamkin DH. Nutritional strategies and growth in extremely low birth weight infants with bronchopulmonary dysplasia over the past 10 years. *J Perinatol.* 2012;32:117–122.
18. Brown LD, Hendrickson K, Masor ML, Hay Jr. WW. High-protein formulas: evidence for use in preterm infants. In: Poindexter B, Karpen H, Jain L, eds. Current concepts in neonatal nutrition. *Clin Perinatol.* 2014;41:383–403.
19. Skinner AM, Battin M, Solimano A, Daaboul J, Kitson HF. Growth and growth factors in premature infants receiving dexamethasone for bronchopulmonary dysplasia. *Amer J Perinatol.* 1997;14:539–546.
20. Jaksic T, Hull MA, Modi B, Ching YA, George D, Compher C; American Society for Parenteral and Enteral Nutrition (A.S.P.E.N.) Board of Directors. A.S.P.E.N. clinical guidelines: Nutrition support of neonates supported with extracorporeal membrane oxygenation. *JPEN J Parenter Enteral Nutr.* 2010;34:247–253.
21. Buck ML, Wooldridge P, Ksenich RA. Comparison of methods of intravenous infusion of fat emulsion during extracorporeal membrane oxygenation. *Pharmacotherapy.* 2005;25:1536–1540.
22. Puangco MA, Schanler RJ. Clinical experience in enteral nutrition support for premature infants with bronchopulmonary dysplasia. *J Perinatol.* 2000;2:87–91.
23. Brunton JA, Saigal S, Atkinson S. Growth and body composition in infants with bronchopulmonary dysplasia up to 3 months corrected age: a randomized trial of a high-energy nutrient-enriched formula fed after hospital discharge. *J Pediatr.* 1998;133:340–345.
24. Bier JA, Ferguson A, Cho C, Oh W, Vohr BR. The oral motor development of low-birth-weight infants who underwent orotracheal intubation during the neonatal period. *Amer J Dis Child.* 1993;147:858–62.
25. Ramanathan R. Bronchopulmonary dysplasia and diuretics. *Neoreviews.* 2008;9:e260–e266.

Chapter 6

Congenital Heart Disease

Emily Trumpower, RD, CSP, CNSC

DISEASE STATE

Congenital heart disease (CHD) occurs in 1% of newborns, who are typically born at full term. Poor energy intake, increased total energy expenditure, malabsorption, and additional medical conditions may be seen depending on the specific defect. Preoperative nutrition and growth is emphasized if the infant needs to reach goal weight before surgery (1).

PREVENTIVE NUTRITION

Nutrition intervention cannot prevent congenital heart defects. In some cases, fluid restriction (≤ 120 mL/kg/d) may prevent congestive heart failure (CHF) in infants with CHD.

TREATMENT NUTRITION

Preoperative Nutrition

Prevent catabolism with sufficient parenteral/enteral energy, protein, and nutrients (see Chapters 2 and 3):

- If the infant is edematous, determine a "dry weight" (often the weight appropriate for length) to calculate nutrition needs **(C)**.

- If fluids are restricted, infuse drip medications in concentrated glucose solutions. Concentrate parenteral nutrition (PN) substrates (glucose, crystalline amino acids [CAA], intravenous fat emulsion [IVFE], and other nutrients) as much as possible **(C)** (1–3).
- Initiate minimal enteral nutrition (MEN), commonly referred to as trophic feeds. Provide 10 to 20 mL/kg/d as MEN unless cyanosis and gut hypoperfusion contraindicate enteral stimulation **(C)**.
- Advance enteral nutrition (EN) as tolerated with concomitant weaning from PN. Use of a standardized feeding protocol for feeding advancement and monitoring of feeding tolerance is recommended for infants whose cardiac lesions are associated with decreased intestinal blood flow, such as hypoplastic left heart, coarctation, and transposition of the great vessels due to increased risk for necrotizing enterocolitis (NEC) **(B)** (1,4).

Promote normal growth for age, normal weight for length, and oral feeding skills:

- Average enteral energy requirements to support growth for both preterm and term infants with CHD are approximately 130 to 150 kcal/kg/d (or 115 kcal/kg/d for ideal body weight for length). Preterm infants, with and without CHD, have higher protein needs, estimated to be 3.5 to 4 g/kg/d. Protein needs of term infants with CHD are less well understood, but they often receive more than the Dietary Reference Intake (DRI) for protein as a result of calorically concentrated feedings and high energy needs (5).
- Allow breastfeeding as tolerated. If needed, provide expressed human milk (ideally hindmilk) and additional nutrients using concentrated liquid formula for term infants and fortification with human milk fortifier (HMF) for preterm infants (< 3.5 kg).

- The use of a supplemental nursing system may allow for breastfeeding while still providing the additional calories and nutrients **(C)**.
- To achieve optimal growth, oral feedings may need to be limited due to the increased energy expenditure that occurs with bottle or breastfeeding. If needed, nasogastric tubes may be used to conserve energy for growth. Nonnutritive sucking or small volume oral feedings should be offered to encourage oral motor development (2).

Postoperative Nutrition

Fluid volume is initially restricted (often to 50 to 80 mL/kg/d); therefore, glucose should be concentrated in drip medications and PN should be concentrated. When evidence of bowel function returns, start with MEN (10 to 20 mL/kg/d) and advance to full feedings in increments of 20 mL/kg/d or as tolerated using a standardized feeding advancement protocol (4).

Rapid postoperative advancement in caloric density of enteral feedings (daily increases from 24 to 27 to 30 kcal/fl oz) is shown to be well tolerated, improve energy intake and weight gain, and result in earlier hospital discharge compared with slower advancement using lower energy-density goals in infants who require staged cardiac surgery later in infancy **(A)** (6).

CHYLOTHORAX

Chylothorax (lymphatic fluid in the chest cavity), either congenital or from operative trauma, is treated nutritionally by limiting the intake of enteral long-chain fatty triglycerides (LCTs) in favor of medium-chain triglycerides (MCTs).

- Provide PN, with IVFE as the source of essential fatty acids (EFAs), and begin MEN with enteral products high in MCT oil when clinically able.
- IVFE can be continued and does not need to be limited. Although IVFE are LCTs, they do not enter the lymphatic system.
- Enfaport (Mead Johnson Nutrition; www.meadjohnson.com) is the only formula with a high MCT oil content (85% of the total fat) that is designed for infants less than 12 months of age, and it is specifically indicated for infants with chylothorax. This product is available only in liquid ready-to-use form, is sterile, and thus is more appropriate for use in infants than the powdered formulas historically used. Formulas containing a lesser percentage of fat content as MCT oil, such as Pregestimil (55% MCT/45% LCT) with added MCT oil, may be considered as transitional feedings as clinical status improves. (See Chapter 3.)
- It is also possible to remove a majority of the fat from human milk and feed the "skimmed" milk to infants with chylothorax (7). Because human milk is not homogenized, this can be done by allowing the fat to separate to the top and then removing the fat. A centrifuge may facilitate this separation (8,9). Additional fortification is required, as "skimmed" milk provides approximately only 10 kcal/oz. Fortification options may include Enfaport ready-to-use liquid, HMF, and/or MCT oil. Water-miscible fat-soluble vitamins may also be given, depending upon the infant's needs. Small amounts of soy oil or other oils rich in linoleic acid and linolenic acid, such as walnut and flax seed oils, respectively, may be added to prevent essential fatty acid deficiency (EFAD) (8).
- To avoid EFAD, feedings should ensure 2% to 4% of calories from LCTs for term infants, For preterm

infants, ensure a linoleic acid intake of 385 to 1,540 mg/kg/d and a linolenic acid intake of > 55 mg/kg/d (10,11). Serum triene:tetraene ratio can be monitored monthly or when clinical symptoms are observed or suspected to drive supplementation strategies.

Nutritional treatment duration is quite variable (averaging 4 to 6 weeks in some centers and 3 to 6 months in others), but should be managed on a case-by-case basis **(C)** (7,12,13). Refractory cases may require medication, surgery, and/or use of PN exclusively until chylous drainage subsides (12,13). If LCTs are limited for greater than 3 months, or if symptoms of EFAD are noted, EFA status can be assessed by measuring the serum triene:tetraene ratio.

PATENT DUCTUS ARTERIOSUS

The ductus arteriosus is a fetal vascular connection that diverts blood from the pulmonary artery to the aorta and placenta for oxygenation. The ductus normally constricts shortly after full-term birth. If it remains open—as it frequently does after preterm birth—it is termed a *patent (open) ductus arteriosus* (PDA).

Incidence is inversely proportional to birth weight and gestational age and occurs in up to 80% in ELBW infants. PDA has the potential to lead to CHF, pulmonary edema, progressive development of pulmonary vascular resistance, and failure to thrive (14).

PDA may close unaided in days or weeks, or may require medical or surgical closure. Infants with a small to moderate PDA can typically start enteral feeding, while infants with a large hemodynamically significant PDA are commonly managed nutritionally with fluid restriction (~120 to 130 mL/kg/d) and concentrated PN.

Medications used to treat PDA, such as ibuprofen and indomethacin, have been thought to decrease intestinal blood flow and increase the risk for NEC (15). However, withholding feeding may actually further decrease mesenteric blood flow and large feeding trials have not demonstrated an increased incidence of NEC with MEN (16,17). Until the PDA is sufficiently closed, fluid restriction is typically necessary, often requiring calorically concentrated feedings, often more than 24 kcal/oz. Once the PDA closes, the infant's enteral feeding plan can be normalized.

REFERENCES

1. Barry JS, Thureen PJ. Nutrition in infants with congenital heart disease. In: Thureen PJ, Hay WW Jr, eds. *Neonatal Nutrition and Metabolism.* 2nd ed. Cambridge, England: Cambridge University Press; 2006:533–542.
2. Cardiac disease. In: Kleinman RE, ed. *American Academy of Pediatrics Pediatric Nutrition Handbook.* 7th ed. Chicago, IL: American Academy of Pediatrics; 2014:1077–1094.
3. Nagle MS and Konek S. Cardiology. In: Samour PQ, King K, eds. *Handbook of Pediatric Nutrition.* 4th ed. Sudbury, MA: Jones and Bartlett Publishers; 2010:313–328.
4. Slicker J, Hehir DA, Horsley M, Monczka J, Stern KW, Roman B, Ocampo EC, Flanagan L, Keenan E, Lambert LM, Davis D, Lamonica M, Rollison N, Heydarian H, Anderson JB; Feeding Work Group of the National Pediatric Cardiology Quality Improvement Collaborative. Nutrition algorithms for infants with hypoplastic left heart syndrome; birth through the first interstage period. *Congenit Heart Dis.* 2013;8:89–102.
5. Steltzer M, Rudd N, and Pick B. Nutrition care for newborns with congenital heart disease. *Clin Perinatol.* 2005;32:1017–1030.
6. Pillo-Blocka F, Adatia I, Sharieff W, McCrindle BW, Zlotkin S. Rapid advancement to more concentrated formula in infants after surgery for congenital heart disease reduces duration of hospital stay: a randomized clinical trial. *J Pediatr.* 2004;145:761–766.
7. Chan GM, Lechtenberg E. The use of fat-free human milk in infants with chylous pleural effusion. *J Perinatol.* 2007;27:434–436.

8. Cox J. Nutrition in neonatal pulmonary disease. In: Dumont RC and Chung Y, eds. *Nutrition in Pediatric Pulmonary Disease*. New York: Humana Press; 2014:55–80.
9. Lessen R. Use of Skim Breast Milk for an Infant with Chylothorax. *ICAN: Infant, Child & Adolescent Nutrition*. 2009;6:303–310.
10. Rodica T. Nutritional approach to pediatric patients with congenital heart defects. *Acta Medica Marisiensis*. 2013;59:121–125.
11. Koletzko B, Poindexter B, Uauy R. In Koletzko B, Poindexter B, Uauy R, eds. Recommended nutrient intake levels for stable, fully enterally fed very low birth weight infants. *Nutritional Care of Preterm Infants: Scientific Basis and Practical Guidelines*. Basel, Switzerland: Karger; 2014:297–299. *World Review of Nutrition and Dietetics*. vol. 110.
12. Chan EH, Russell JL, Williams WG, Van Arsdell GS, Coles JG, McCrindle BW. Postoperative chylothorax after cardiothoracic surgery in children. *Ann Thorac Surg*. 2005;80:1864–1870.
13. Densupsoontorn NS, Jirapinyo P, Wongarn R, Thamonsiri N, Nana A, Laohaprasitiporn D, Soongswang J, Durongpisitkul KD, Pornvilawan SA. Management of chylothorax and chylopericardium in pediatric patients: experiences at Siriraj Hospital, Bangkok. *Asia Pac J Clin Nutr*. 2005;14:182–187.
14. Poole-Napp E. Patent ductus arteriosus. In: Groh-Wargo S, Thompson M, Cox JH, eds. *Nutritional Care for High-Risk Newborns*. 3rd ed. Chicago, IL: Precept Press; 2000:391–396.
15. Coombs RC, Morgan MEI, Durbin GM, et al. Gut blood flow velocities in the newborn: effects of patent ductus arteriosus and parenteral indomethacin. *Arch Dis Child*. 1990;65:1067.
16. Neu J. In Koletzko B, Poindexter B, Uauy R, eds. Necrotizing enterocolitis. *Nutritional Care of Preterm Infants: Scientific Basis and Practical Guidelines*. Basel, Switzerland: Karger; 2014:253–263. *World Review of Nutrition and Dietetics*. vol. 110.
17. Clymen R, Wickremasinghe A, Jhaveri N, Hassinger DC, Attridge JT, Sanocka U, Polin R, Gillam-Krakauer M, Reese J, Mammel M, Couser R, Mulrooney N, Yanowitz TD, Derrick M, Jegatheesan P, Walsh M, Fujii A, Porta N, Carey WA, Swanson JR; Ductus Arteriosus Feed or Fast with Indomethacin or Ibuprofen (DAFFII) Investigators. Enteral feeding during indomethacin and ibuprofen treatment of a patent ductus arteriousus. *J Pediatr*. 2013;163:406–411.

Chapter 7

Necrotizing Enterocolitis

Michelle Johnson, RD, CSP, LD

DISEASE STATE

Necrotizing enterocolitis (NEC) is an acquired, life-threatening gastrointestinal disease often associated with feeding. Overall incidence in the United States is between 3% and 10% in very low birth weight (VLBW) infants and is inversely related to gestational age (GA) (1). Pathophysiology is believed to be multifactorial (see Figure 7.1) (2). Risk factors include prematurity, enteral feedings, bowel ischemia, abnormal bacterial colonization, and polycythemia.

Manifestations include the following:

- Systemic: temperature instability, lethargy, apnea, bradycardia, tachycardia, hypotension / hypotensive shock
- Gastrointestinal: poor feeding, increasing residuals, emesis, abdominal distension and/or tenderness, abdominal wall discoloration, ileus with decreased bowel sounds, occult or grossly bloody stools (no fissure).

Figure 7.1 Pathophysiology of Necrotizing Enterocolitis

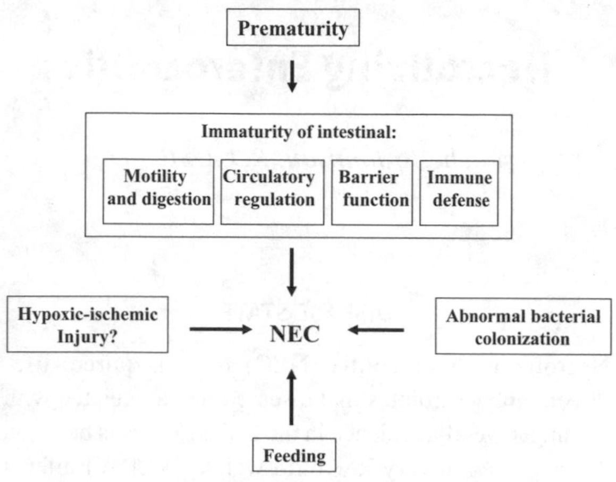

Source: Reprinted from Lin PW, Stoll BJ. Necrotising enterocolitis. *The Lancet.* 2006;368:1271–1283, with permission of Elsevier.

Infants are categorized by Bell et al's stages for NEC (3): stage I: suspected; stage II: definite; stage III: advanced disease, with pneumatosis intestinalis or portal venous gas on abdominal x-ray as diagnostic radiologic signs of NEC. Modifications of the Bell staging classifications are in use (4).

PREVENTIVE NUTRITION

Although enteral nutrition (EN) is a risk factor for development of NEC, not all infants in whom NEC develops have been fed enterally (5). Withholding feedings in the first few days after birth has not been shown to be protective against NEC and should be carefully weighed against the potential positive effects of luminal nutrients on gastrointestinal, endocrine, and metabolic maturity (6).

Common nutrition practices proposed to reduce the incidence of NEC include the following (7–13):

- Human milk: widely accepted as the most effective way to reduce NEC **(A)**. Fortification of human milk is standard of care for preterm infants and is not associated with a significant difference in risk of NEC compared with unfortified human milk feedings **(B)**. If mother's own milk is unavailable and donor human milk is accessible, donor human milk should be considered as an alternative to formula **(B)**. While meta-analysis of studies including infants fed donor human milk detected a significantly lower incidence of NEC compared with infants fed formula **(B)**, further studies assessing this effect using donor milk with a commercially available human milk fortifier (HMF) are indicated. A diet of human milk fortified with human milk–based fortifier is associated with lower NEC compared with bovine-based milk products **(B)**.
- Development and use of a standardized approach to feeding **(A)**.

Feeding practices likely to have no effect on occurrence of NEC include the following **(A)** (6,14–18):

- Minimal enteral nutrition (MEN) vs enteral fasting **(B)**. Infants who receive MEN tolerate full feedings faster and have a shorter length of hospital stay. A.S.P.E.N. guidelines state to begin MEN within the first 2 days of life.
- Early (≤ 4 days of life) vs late (days of life 6 to 10) advancement of feedings beyond 24 mL/kg/d **(A)**
- Rate of feeding advancement by 30 to 35 mL/kg/d compared with 15 to 20 mL/kg/d **(A)**
- Bolus vs continuous feeding **(A)**

- A potentially harmful nutrition practice that may increase NEC is pharmacological supplemental vitamin E that results in serum levels > 3.5 mg/dL **(A)** (19). While enteral probiotic supplementation for infants with birth weight > 1,000 g has been shown to reduce the incidence of severe NEC **(B)** (20); optimal probiotic strain(s), availability, dose, duration of therapy, and safety remain to be determined. Due to a lack of safety data, the FDA recommends caution in applying the science of dietary probiotic supplementation in clinical practice (21).

Efforts to increase the availability of fresh "own mother's milk" are perhaps the best strategy to minimize the risk of NEC (22,23).

TREATMENT NUTRITION

Management of NEC includes antibiotic therapy and support of physiological homeostasis. There is no known optimal nutritional management during active or recovering NEC, but consider the following strategies **(C)**:

- Balanced and complete total parenteral nutrition (TPN) (see Chapter 2, Parenteral Nutrition), with cessation of EN for bowel rest, ranging in clinical practice from days to weeks. Infants with subclinical NEC may recover within several days of feeding cessation, cautious reinitiation, and provision of supportive care (1). Reinitiation of feedings at a median of 4 days, compared with a median of 10 days, following diagnosis of Bell's stage II or greater NEC revealed less time to achieve full feedings, less catheter-related sepsis, and shorter length of hospital stay (24).
- Gradual reintroduction of enteral feedings as tolerated: increase by 10 to 35 mL/kg/d with human milk

(preferred), donor human milk or preterm formula (if mother's own milk is not available), or protein hydrolysate or amino acid–based formula (if evidence of intolerance to intact protein is present).

- After NEC resolves, preterm infants who resume feedings with human milk require fortification. Options include gradual introduction of commercial HMF to a concentration of 1 packet per 25 mL (goal), fortification with donor human milk–based human milk fortifier, or with specific nutrients (if intolerant to commercial fortifier options) (see Chapter 3, Enteral Nutrition).
- Bowel injury and prolonged gut rest may precipitate secondary intestinal enzyme deficiencies; anticipate and treat feeding intolerance with individualized enteral feedings and/or feedings built from modular products.
- If bowel resection is necessary, carefully review nutrients that may be maldigested/malabsorbed.
- Monitor for late complications such as cholestatic jaundice (when TPN is administered for more than 2 weeks), bowel strictures (manifested by sudden or increasing gastric residuals and/or emesis), and osteopenia (see Chapter 15, Osteopenia of Prematurity).

REFERENCES

1. Clark DA, Munshi UK. Feeding associated neonatal necrotizing enterocolitis (Primary NEC) is an inflammatory bowel disease. *Pathophysiology*. 2014;21:29–34.
2. Lin PW, Stoll BJ. Necrotising enterocolitis. *Lancet*. 2006;368:1271–1283.
3. Bell MJ, Ternberg JL, Feigin RD, Keating JP, Marshall R, Barton L, Brotherthon T. Neonatal necrotizing enterocolitis: therapeutic decisions based on clinical staging. *Ann Surg*. 1978;187:1–7

4. Walsh MC, Kleigman RM. Necrotizing enterocolitis: treatment based on staging criteria. *Pediatr Clins North Am.* 1986;33:179–201.
5. Srinivasan PS, Brandler MD, D'Souza A. Necrotizing enterocolitis. *Clin Perinatol.* 2008;35:251–272.
6. Morgan J, Bombell S, McGuire W. Early trophic feeding versus enteral fasting for very preterm or very low birth weight infants. *Cochrane Database Syst Rev.* 2013;(3): CD000504.
7. Cristofalo EA, Schanler RJ, Blanco CL, Sullivan S, Trawoeger R, Kiechl-Kohlendorfer U et al. Randomized trial of exclusive human milk versus preterm formula diets in extremely premature infants. *J Pediatr*. 2013;163:1592–1595.
8. Kuschel CA, Harding JE. Multicomponent fortified human milk for promoting growth in preterm infants. *Cochrane Database Syst Rev.* 2004;(1):CD000343.
9. Herrmann K, Carroll K. An exclusively human milk diet reduces necrotizing enterocolitis. *Breastfeed Med.* 2014;9:184–190.
10. Patole S. Prevention and treatment of necrotizing enterocolitis in preterm neonates. *Early Hum Dev.* 2007;83:635–642.
11. Quigley M, McGuire W. Formula versus donor breast milk for feeding preterm or low birth weight infants. *Cochrane Database Syst Rev.* 2014;(4):CD002971.
12. Section on Breastfeeding. Breastfeeding and the use of human milk. *Peds*. 2012;129:e827–e841.
13. Sullivan S, Schanler RJ, Kim JH, Patel AL, Trawoger R, Kiechl-Kohlendorfer U, Chan GM, Blanco CL, Abrams S, Cotten CM, Laroia N, Ehrenkranz RA, Dudell G, Cristofalo EA, Meier P, Lee ML, Rechtman DJ, Lucas A. An exclusively human milk-based diet is associated with a lower rate of necrotizing enterocolitis than a diet of human milk and bovine milk-based products. *J Pediatr*. 2010;156:562–567.
14. Nectrotizing Enterocolitis (NEC) Guideline Team, Cincinnati Children's Hospital Medical Center. Evidence-based care guideline for necrotizing enterocolitis (NEC) among very low birth weight infants. Pediatric Evidence-Based Care Guidelines, Cincinnati Children's Hospital Medical Center Guideline 28. 2010:1–10.
15. Fallon EM, Deepika N, Potemkin AK, Gura KM, Simpser E, Compher C; American Society for Parenteral and Enteral Nutrition (A.S.P.E.N.) Board of Directors, Puder M. A.S.P.E.N. Clinical Guidelines: Nutrition support of neonatal patients at

risk for necrotizing enterocolitis. *JPEN J Parenter Enteral Nutr.* 2012;36:506–523.

16. Morgan J, Young L, McGuire W. Delayed introduction of progressive enteral feeds to prevent necrotising enterocolitis in very low birth weight infants. *Cochrane Database Syst Rev.* 2011;(3):CD001970.
17. Morgan J, Young L, McGuire W. Slow advancement of enteral feed volumes to prevent necrotising enterocolitis in very low birth weight infants. *Cochrane Database Syst Rev.* 2011;(3):CD001241.
18. Premji SS, Chessell L. Continuous nasogastric milk feeding versus intermittent bolus milk feeding for premature infants less than 1500 grams. *Cochrane Database Syst Rev.* 2011;(11):CD001819.
19. Brion LP, Bell EF, Raghuveer TS. Vitamin E supplementation for prevention of morbidity and mortality in preterm infants. *Cochrane Database Syst Rev*. 2003;(4):CD003665.
20. AlFaleh K, Anabrees J. Probiotics for prevention of necrotizing enterocolitis in preterm infants. *Cochrane Database Syst Rev.* 2014;(4):CD005496. doi: 10.1002/14651858.CD005496.pub4.
21. Center for Biologics Evaluation and Research, Center for Food Safety and Applied Nutrition. *Important Drug Warning Regarding Use of Dietary Supplements in Immunocompromised Persons.* December 9, 2014. http://www.fda.gov/downloads/BiologicsBloodVaccines/SafetyAvailability/UCM426233.pdf. Accessed March 23, 2015.
22. Lee HC, Kurtin PS, Wight NE, Chance K, Cucinotta-Fobes T, Hanson-Timpson TA, Nisbet CC, Rhine WD, Risingsun K, Wood M, Danielsen BH, Sharek PJ. A quality improvement project to increase breast milk use in very low birth weight infants. *Pediatrics*. 2012;130:e1679–e1687.
23. Renfrew MJ, Dyson L, McCormick F, Misso K, Stenhouse E, King SE, Williams AF. Breastfeeding promotion for infants in neonatal units: a systematic review. *Child Care Health Dev.* 2009;36:165–178.
24. Bohnhort B, Müller S, Dŏrdelmann M, Peter CS, Petersen C, Poets CF. Early feeding after necrotizing enterocolitis in preterm infants. *J Pediatr*. 2003;143:484–487.

Chapter 8

Short Bowel Syndrome

Michelle Johnson, RD, CSP, LD

DISEASE STATE

Short bowel syndrome (SBS) is defined functionally as malabsorption in conjunction with a shortened bowel length. Intestinal failure describes malabsorption of intestinal contents that is inadequate to maintain growth, hydration, and/or electrolyte homeostasis.

The most common reason for SBS in the neonatal intensive care unit (NICU) is necrotizing enterocolitis (NEC), followed by congenital malformations (eg, gastroschisis, intestinal atresia) and volvulus (1). Overall, the incidence of SBS is 25 per 100,000 live births and is much more common in preterm, rather than term, infants (2). Incidence is 7 per 1,000 very low birth weight (VLBW) infants, and 11 per 1,000 extremely low birth weight (ELBW) infants (1). Mortality can approach 40% (2).

Residual bowel length and function, region of bowel remaining, etiology of SBS, and age of the patient are used to guide and anticipate response to treatment. See Figure 8.1 for sites of gastrointestinal tract absorption and secretion.

Figure 8.1 Sites of Gastrointestinal Absorption and Secretion

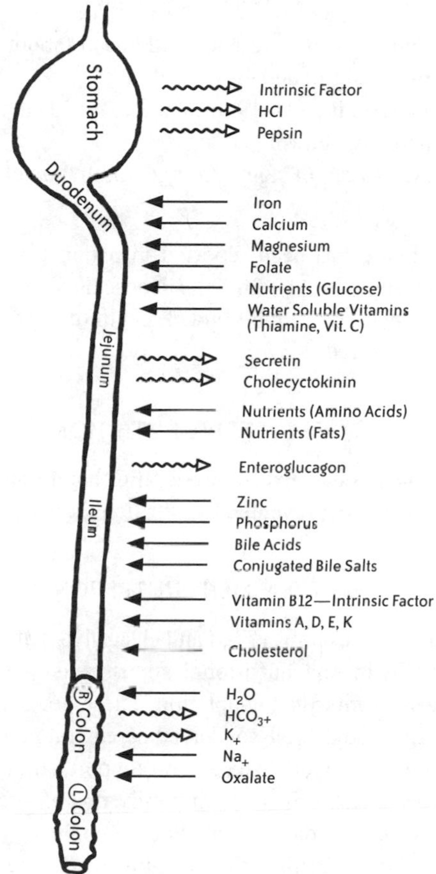

Source: This figure was published in Clinics in Perinatology, vol 21(2), Ricketts RR, Surgical treatment of necrotizing enterocolitis and the short bowel syndrome, 365–387, Copyright Elsevier 1994.

The following estimates of bowel length are used to guide and anticipate response to treatment:

- Term infants: 240-cm small bowel (about five times birth length) and 40-cm colon
- Preterm infants (19 to 27 weeks): 150 cm total small and large bowel
- At 1 year of age, average small bowel length is 380 cm

Survival has been reported in patients with a small bowel length of ≤ 15 cm if the ileocecal valve is intact and in patients with a small bowel length of > 15 cm but no ileocecal valve (3).

PREVENTIVE NUTRITION

With the possible exception of NEC, conditions resulting in SBS are not prevented by nutrition therapy.

TREATMENT NUTRITION

Goals are to establish fluid and electrolyte balance, maintain growth and nutritional status, and maximize the process of intestinal adaptation. These goals are accomplished through well-conceived parenteral nutrition (PN) regimens, individualized enteral support, strict adherence to procedures designed to minimize risk of infection, and experienced medical/surgical management.

Specific nutrition therapy guidelines are primarily based on accumulated clinical experience of practitioners (lowest level of evidence-based practice) **(C)** (3).

Parenteral Nutrition

In addition to the PN goals discussed in Chapter 2, PN goals for infants with SBS are as follows:

- Minimize total parenteral nutrition (TPN)–associated cholestasis by avoiding excessive calories. Lipid restriction to 1 gm/kg per day, compared with 2.5 to 3 gm/kg per day, has resulted in significantly lower direct bilirubin levels (4,5). Close monitoring of growth with an increase in the glucose infusion rate to meet parenteral energy needs, and screening for essential fatty acid deficiency (EFAD) should accompany this practice. Monitor trace elements, including:
    - Copper: Monitor copper and ceruloplasmin levels. Consider reducing copper only if evidence of copper toxicity is detected (6), or reducing copper to 10 mcg/kg/d if direct bilirubin is > 2 mg/dL.
    - Manganese: remove completely if direct bilirubin is > 2 mg/dL.
    - Zinc: consider providing > 400 mcg/kg/d if significant ostomy or stool losses are present.
- For infants who can reasonably tolerate a temporary cessation of a continuous supply of parenteral glucose, consider cycling off PN for 2 to 4 hours per day to decrease the incidence or delay the onset of cholestasis (7).

Enteral Nutrition (EN)

Goals for EN include the following:

- Schedule: Initiate trophic feedings at 10 to 15 mL/kg per day postoperatively once signs and symptoms of bowel function are present and continue for several days; slowly increase volume by ~10 mL/kg per day as tolerated.

- Composition: Mother's own colostrum and milk (donor milk is not known to offer the same advantages of mother's own milk), extensively hydrolyzed protein formula, or amino acid–based formula (preferred over extensively hydrolyzed protein formulas by some because of theoretical risk of secondary non-IgE-mediated intestinal allergic disease in patients with SBS). A dual source of fats in formula is beneficial, as long-chain triglycerides (LCTs) promote intestinal adaptation but are not as well absorbed as medium-chain triglycerides (MCTs) (8). Due to the potential for lactose malabsorption, a formula that contains glucose polymers as its primary carbohydrate source may be beneficial (8). Ideal feeding composition has not yet been determined (9).
- Route of administration: Initially, use continuous enteral feeding by oro/nasogastric (short-term), gastrostomy (long-term), or transpyloric patients (those with poor gastric emptying). With gastric feedings, gradually transition to bolus/intermittent feedings. Offer nonnutritive sucking and small-volume oral feedings several times per day, as tolerated, to avoid feeding aversion (10).
- Micronutrients: Monitor micronutrient status with special attention to fat-soluble vitamins A, D, E, and K (if fat malabsorption is present); trace elements (especially iron and zinc); calcium, phosphorus, and magnesium (particularly in preterm infants); and vitamin B-12 after terminal ileal resection (11).

Supplement routinely with multivitamins; consider water-miscible, fat-soluble vitamins if fat malabsorption and/or cholestasis are present; consider intramuscular delivery of vitamin B-12 and vitamin K; consider additional zinc for wound healing and to account for gastrointestinal tract losses.

Response to Treatment

The goals of treatment are little or no vomiting, growth at expected rate for age, and normal nutritional biochemical levels. Feeding volume can be advanced gradually until daily stool output threshold is reached. As bowel adaptation occurs, further volume or caloric density changes can be introduced (9). The presence of reducing substances in the stool and/or acidic stool contents suggests carbohydrate malabsorption. Thus, stool/ostomy output guidelines include the following (11):

- Volume ≤ 50 mL/kg/d
- Negative reducing substances in the stool
- Stool pH ≥ 5.5 (applies to infants with intact colon)

For feeding intolerance manifested as excessive stool/ostomy output, consider discontinuing feeding volume advancements, returning to most recently tolerated feeding volume or caloric density, or changing to continuous feedings. Prior to and during enteral feeding, monitor fluid and electrolyte status and replace losses from drainage or feeding tubes, or stool/ostomy if output is excessive (see Table 8.1) (12). Consider measuring serum zinc if stool or ileostomy fluid losses are significant. Zinc content of stool output is approximately 12 to 17 mg/L (12).

Table 8.1 Gastrointestinal Electrolyte Losses

	Sodium, mEq/L	Potassium, mEq/L	Chloride, mEq/L	Bicarbonate, mEq/L
Gastric	140	15	155	—
Ileostomy	80–140	15	115	40
Colostomy	50–80	10–30	40	20–25
Secretory	60–120	—	—	—
Diarrhea	30–40	10–80	10–110	30
Normal stool	5	10	10	0

Source: Adapted with permission from Wessel JJ: Short bowel syndrome. In: Groh-Wargo S, Thompson M, Cox JH, eds. *Nutritional Care of High Risk Newborns*. Chicago, IL: Precept Press; 2000:469.

Additional Treatment Options

- Refeeding of proximal enterostomy effluent into a mucous fistula can stimulate bowel adaptation (13) and reduce development of intestinal atrophy in the distal portion of the gastrointestinal tract (14).
- Soluble fiber may reduce diarrhea and enhance intestinal adaptation. Sources include liquid fruit pectin (eg, Certo, Kraft Foods) (1% to 3% or 1 to 3 mL per 100 mL formula) (3) or partially hydrolyzed guar gum (1 g per 40 mL formula). Use cautiously in the presence of bacterial overgrowth.
- Medications. Gastric acid suppression medications such as ranitidine may prevent hypersecretion. Motility agents such as loperamide may slow intestinal transit. Antimicrobial drugs (metronidazole) are indicated to treat bacterial overgrowth. Additional medications that may be indicated include octreotide to decrease stool output, ursodiol to decrease

cholestasis, and cholestyramine to decrease bile acids in the colon (10).

- A systematic review of probiotic use in infants and children with SBS revealed common complications of probiotic sepsis and D-lactic acidosis, with insufficient evidence to inform practice at this time (15). Due to a lack of safety data, the FDA recommends caution in applying the science of dietary probiotic supplementation in clinical practice. (16).

Continuing Care

Sudden, unexplained abdominal distention and/or vomiting may signal the development of intestinal strictures requiring surgical intervention (10). Introduction of solid foods is usually recommended after 4 to 6 months corrected age and helps to maintain oral-motor skills. Starches, vegetables, and meats are likely to be better tolerated than simple sugars, fruit juices, and lactose-containing foods. Green beans as a source of fiber may improve bowel function (3,11).

REFERENCES

1. Cole CR, Hansen NI, Higgins RD, Ziegler TR, Stoll BJ. Very low birth weight preterm infants with surgical short bowel syndrome: incidence, morbidity and mortality, and growth outcomes at 18 to 22 months. *Pediatrics*. 2008;122:e573–e582.
2. Wales PW, de Silva N, Kim J, Lecce L, To T, Moore A. Neonatal short bowel syndrome: population-based estimates of incidence and mortality rates. *J Pediatr Surg.* 2004;39:690–695.
3. Wessel JJ, Kocoshis SA. Nutritional management of infants with short bowel syndrome. *Semin Perinatol.* 2007;31:104–111.
4. Sanchez SE, Braun LP, Mercer LD, Sherrill M, Stevens J, Javid PJ. The effect of lipid restriction on the prevention of parenteral nutrition-associated cholestasis in surgical infants. *J Pediatr Surg*. 2013;48:573–578.

5. Rollins MD, Ward RM, Jackson WD, Mulroy CW, Spencer CP, Ying J, Greene T, Book LS. Effect of decreased soybean lipid emulsion on hepatic function in infants at risk for parenteral nutrition-associated liver disease: a pilot study. *J Pediatr Surg.* 2013;48:1348–1356.
6. Blackmer AB and Bailey E. Management of copper deficiency in cholestatic infants: review of the literature and a case series. *Nutr Clin Pract.* 2013;28:75–86.
7. Jensen AR, Goldin AB, Koopmeiners JS, Stevens J, Waldhausen JHT, Kim SS. The association of cyclic parenteral nutrition and decreased incidence of cholestatic liver disease in patients with gastroschisis. *J Pediatr Surg*. 2009;44:183–189.
8. Batra AB, Beattie RM. Management of short bowel syndrome in infancy. *Early Hum Dev*. 2013;89:899–904.
9. Amin SC, Pappas C, Iyengar H, Maheshwari A. Short bowel syndrome in the NICU. *Clin Perinatol*. 2013;40:53–68.
10. Hwang ST, Schulman RJ. Update on management and treatment of short gut. *Clin Perinatol.* 2002;29:181–194.
11. Serrano MS, Schmidt-Sommerfeld E. Nutrition support of infants with short bowel syndrome. *Nutrition.* 2002;18:966–970.
12. Wessel JJ. Short bowel syndrome. In: Groh-Wargo S, Thompson M, Cox JH, eds. *Nutritional Care of High Risk Newborns.* Chicago, IL: Precept Press; 2000:469.
13. Richardson L, Banerjee S, Rabe H. What is the evidence on the practice of mucous fistula refeeding in neonates with short bowel syndrome? *J Pediatr Gastroenterol Nutr.* 2006;43:267–270.
14. Drenckpohl D, Vegunta R, Knaub L, Holterman M, Wang H, Macwan K, Pearl R. Reinfusion of succus entericus into the mucous fistula decreases dependence on parenteral nutrition in neonates. *ICAN: Infant, Child, & Adolescent Nutrition.* 2012;4:168–174.
15. Reddy VS, Patole SK, Rao S. Role of probiotics in short bowel syndrome in infants and children—a systematic review. *Nutrients*. 2013;5:679–699.
16. Center for Biologics Evaluation and Research, Center for Food Safety and Applied Nutrition. *Important Drug Warning Regarding Use of Dietary Supplements in Immunocompromised Persons.* December 9, 2014. http://www.fda.gov/downloads/BiologicsBloodVaccines/SafetyAvailability/UCM426233.pdf. Accessed March 23, 2015.

Chapter 9

Hyperbilirubinemia

Amy Gates, RD, CSP, LD

DISEASE STATE

Hyperbilirubinemia is a symptom, not a specific disease. Unconjugated (indirect) bilirubin levels may become elevated within the first week of life as a result of increased breakdown of red blood cells, or due to enhanced enterohepatic recirculation of bilirubin caused by decreased intestinal motility or intestinal obstruction, or a combination of both. Medical treatment is not required unless serum bilirubin concentration reaches levels that place the infant at increased risk for neurologic damage (kernicterus). Breastfed infants may present with a second or late form of unconjugated hyperbilirubinemia, which occurs beyond the first or second week of life, particularly if stools are infrequent.

Elevated levels of conjugated (direct) bilirubin indicate compromised liver function. Conjugated hyperbilirubinemia occurs with diseases that prevent excretion of bile from the liver by obstruction or hepatic tissue injury, including neonatal hepatitis, biliary atresia, primary biliary cirrhosis, metabolic disorders, or cholestasis associated with prolonged parenteral nutrition (PN).

PREVENTIVE NUTRITION

Unconjugated Hyperbilirubinemia

Breastfed infants are more likely to become jaundiced than formula-fed infants are. The increased risk is associated with lower volume intake resulting in weight loss (1,2). Evidence of adequate intake in breastfed infants is 4 to 6 wet diapers in 24 hours and the passage of 3 to 4 stools per day by the fourth day of life (3). Encourage 9 to 12 feedings per day of human milk or formula to promote adequate hydration and intestinal motility. Supplementation of breastfed infants with water does not prevent or improve elevated bilirubin levels **(A)** (4–9).

Conjugated Hyperbilirubinemia

Although nutrition strategies to prevent the occurrence of inborn errors of metabolism do not exist, nutrition therapies for prevention of hepatic damage due to inborn errors of metabolism have been described elsewhere (9). Nutrition-related strategies that may decrease risk or severity of cholestasis associated with PN include the following:

- Provide adequate, but not excessive, macronutrients. Meet protein needs for age and clinical condition, providing 60% to 70% of nonprotein calories as carbohydrate and 30% to 40% of nonprotein calories as fat **(B)** (5–9).
- Consider cyclic administration of PN **(C)**. (See Chapter 2.) Cycling of PN may not be appropriate for the preterm infant or term infants under 3 months of age.
- Use pediatric amino acid preparations containing taurine, especially for preterm infants or infants in whom necrotizing enterocolitis (NEC) develops **(B)** (5–9).

- A new parenteral lipid emulsion, Omegaven, containing primarily n-3 fatty acids and made from fish oils, may be a promising alternative product to prevent cholestasis **(C)**. Omegaven is currently approved for use in Europe, but approved only for compassionate use in the United States. Research is currently underway to seek Food and Drug Administration approval of this product (10).
- Introduce and advance enteral feedings as soon as possible **(A)** (3–7).
- Restriction of intravenous soy-based lipids to 1 g/kg/d in PN-fed surgical infants has been associated with a reduction in the incidence of liver disease, but studies reported to date are not large, randomized, controlled trials. In light of the negative effect of early growth deficits on developmental outcomes, growth should be carefully monitored, and lipid doses increased when needed to support normal growth. Serum triene:tetraene ratios should be monitored so that lipid dose can be increased as needed to ensure adequate essential fatty acid status, although this does not ensure adequate very-long-chain fatty acid status (11–14).

TREATMENT NUTRITION

Unconjugated Hyperbilirubinemia

If bilirubin levels increase to > 20 mg/dL in infants with breast milk jaundice, discontinue breastfeeding for 24 to 48 hours and provide infant formula instead during this time. Counsel the mother about how to promote maintenance of breast milk supply and when to resume breastfeeding **(C)** (3,6). Expression of mother's milk during this cessation, by hand or with a breast pump, is necessary to maintain lactation.

Conjugated Hyperbilirubinemia

Consider the following during administration of PN:

- Tactics to prevent cholestasis should be continued (see Preventive Nutrition earlier in this chapter) (3–10).
- When enteral feedings are tolerated, consider use of ursodeoxycholic acid, which has been shown to reduce cholestasis by increasing bile flow **(B)** (7,8).
- Although copper is excreted in bile, hepatic levels of copper decrease as liver disease progresses, and copper deficiency has developed in pediatric patients when copper is removed from parenteral solutions. Reduce or remove copper only if evidence of copper toxicity is present **(C)** (15,16).
- Manganese is also excreted primarily in bile, but blood manganese levels are elevated in patients with cholestatic jaundice and are directly correlated to level of cholestasis. At this time, it seems appropriate to remove manganese from PN when direct bilirubin is > 2 mg/dL. Excessive intakes of parenteral manganese may induce PN-associated liver disease and neurotoxicity **(C)** (17).
- Case reports using a new parenteral lipid emulsion containing primarily n-3 fatty acids made from fish oils (Omegaven; not currently approved for use in the United States) also show resolution of cholestatic jaundice **(C)** (10).

The following are considerations with enteral feedings:

- Energy needs may be 125% of the normal recommended amounts based on ideal body weight (5–8).

- Medium-chain triglycerides (MCTs) do not require bile salts for absorption. Formula with MCT oil may be used, but the formula should also provide adequate amounts of oils rich in linoleic and linolenic acids to prevent EFA deficiency (5–8). Preterm infant formulas contain a substantial amount of MCT oil as well as oils rich in EFAs. Chapter 3 (Enteral Nutrition) lists types of term formulas that contain substantial amounts of MCT oil **(C)**.
- If stools appear acholic (without bile; usually white, grey, or clay-colored) or if fat malabsorption is present, obtain serum levels of fat-soluble vitamins A, D, and E and prothrombin time or PIVKA II to assess vitamin K status **(C)**. Box 9.1 lists recommendations for supplementation of fat-soluble vitamins (5–8,18–24).
- Recommended oral intake of water-soluble vitamins is twice the Recommended Dietary Allowance **(C)**.
- Reduced bile salt presence in the bowel may cause steatorrhea, which may in turn affect absorption of minerals. Maintain optimal intake of calcium, phosphorus, and zinc **(C)** (6).

Box 9.1 Recommendations for Supplementation of Vitamins A, E, D, and K in Enteral Nutrition Therapy for Conjugated Hyperbilirubinemia[a]

Vitamin A

- Supplement with enteral/oral doses of 5,000 to 25,000 IU/d in water-miscible form as needed to prevent deficiency. Serum levels of < 20 mcg/L indicate deficiency.
- Monitor for signs of toxicity. Serum levels > 100 mcg/dL identify potential toxicity.

(continued)

Box 9.1 Recommendations for Supplementation of Vitamins A, E, D, and K in Enteral Nutrition Therapy for Conjugated Hyperbilirubinemia[a] (continued)

Vitamin E

- Supplement with enteral/oral doses of 50 to 400 IU/d in water-miscible form or 15 to 25 IU/kg/d as d-alpha-tocopherol polyethylene glycol-1,000 succinate to prevent deficiency. Serum levels < 0.5 mg/dL indicate deficiency.
- Higher doses, or doses that support serum levels >3.5 mg/dL, have been associated with an increased incidence of NEC, possibly due to the high osmolality of the preparation; such doses may cause diarrhea or exacerbate vitamin K–deficiency coagulopathy.
- Serum levels > 5 mg/dL are associated with increased incidence of sepsis.

Vitamin D

- Vitamin D levels < 20 ng/mL may be considered evidence of vitamin D deficiency, and levels between 21 and 29 ng/mL may be considered evidence of insufficiency. Hypophosphatemia (serum phosphorus < 4 mg/dL) may also be present, as may hypocalcemia (serum calcium level < 8 mg/dL). Alkaline phosphatase levels may be elevated to > 600 IU/L.
- To maintain normal vitamin D levels in infants with cholestasis, provide enteral/oral dose of 400 to 1,000 IU/d cholecalciferol.
- If there is evidence of insufficiency or deficiency, supplement with enteral/oral doses of 2,500 to 8,000 IU/d of D-2 ergocalciferol or 2 to 4 mcg/kg/d 25-hydroxyvitamin D.
- Calcium (25 to 100 mg/kg/d) and phosphorus (25 to 50 mg/kg/d) supplements may also be needed if rickets or osteomalacia is present. When supplementing with calcium and phosphorus, monitor serum levels every 10 to 14 days.
- Monitor serum 25(OH)D concentrations every 30 days during supplementation, as vitamin D toxicity is rare but may cause hypercalcemia, hypercalciuria and/or nephrocalcinosis.

(continued)

Box 9.1 (continued)

Vitamin K

- 2.5 to 5 mg every 2 to 3 days.
- Measuring serum levels of phylloquinone or vitamin K–dependent protein PIVKA-II is used to detect subclinical deficiency and is a more sensitive indicator of vitamin K status. Coagulation studies are often used as a surrogate marker when PIVKA II and/or phylloquinone are not available. Restoration of a normal prothrombin time (PT) after vitamin K administration confirms deficiency.

[a]Fat-soluble vitamin deficiencies are more likely to occur when serum total serum bilirubin levels are > 2 mg/dL. Although multivitamin preparations using water-miscible forms of the fat-soluble vitamins may be used, they do not guarantee fat-soluble vitamin sufficiency. Consistent monitoring is recommended to drive additional vitamin supplementation strategies (18).
Source: Data are from references 5–8 and 18–24.

REFERENCES

1. Chang RJ, Chou HC, Chang YH, Chen MH, Chen CY, Hsieh WS, Tsao PN. Weight loss percentage prediction of subsequent neonatal hyperbilirubinemia in exclusively breastfed neonates. *Pediatr Neonatol.* 2012;53:41–44.
2. Flaherman VJ, Schaefer EW, Kuzniewicz MW, Li SX, Walsh EM, Paul IM. Early weight loss nomograms for exclusively breastfed newborns. *Pediatrics.* 2015;135:e16–e23.
3. American Academy of Pediatrics. Management of hyperbilirubinemia in the newborn infant 35 weeks' gestation or more. *Pediatrics* 2004;114:297–316.
4. Askin DF, Diehl-Jones WL. The neonatal liver part III: pathophysiology of liver dysfunction. *Neonatal Netw.* 2003;22:5–15.
5. Gourley GR. Breastfeeding, diet, and neonatal hyperbilirubinemia. *Pediatr Rev Neo Rev.* 2000;1:e25–e31.
6. Hartline JV. Hyperbilirubinemia. In: Groh-Wargo S, Thompson M, Cox JH, eds. *Nutritional Care for High-Risk Newborns.* 3rd ed. Chicago, IL: Precept Press; 2000:409–424.

7. Venigalla S, Gourley GR. Neonatal cholestasis. *Semin Perinatol.* 2004;28:348–355.
8. Francavilla R, Miniello VL, Brunetti L, Lionetti ME, Armenio L. Hepatitis and cholestasis in infancy: clinical and nutritional aspects. *Acta Paediatr Suppl.* 2003;441:101–104.
9. Acosta P, Yannicelli S. *The Ross Metabolic Formula System: Nutrition Support Protocols.* 4th ed. Columbus, OH: Ross Products Division/Abbott Laboratories; 2001.
10. Gura KM, Duggan CP, Collier SB, Jennings RW, Folkman J, Bistrian BR, Puder M. Reversal of parenteral nutrition–associated liver disease in two infants with short bowel syndrome using parenteral fish oil: implications for future management. *Pediatrics.* 2006;118:e197–e201.
11. Sanchez S, Braun LP, Mercer LD, Sherrill M, Stevens J, Javid PJ. The effect of lipid restriction on the prevention of parenteral nutrition-associated cholestasis in surgical infants. *J Pediatr Surg.* 2013;48:573–578.
12. Cober MP, Killu G, Brattain A, Welch KB, Kunisaki SM, Teitelbaum DH. Intravenous fat emulsions reduction for patients with parenteral nutrition-associated liver disease. *J Pediatr.* 2012;160:421–427.
13. Jakobsen MS, Jorgensen MH, Husby S, Andersen L, Jeppesen PB. Low fat high carbohydrate parenteral nutrition may potentially reverse liver disease in long term PN dependent infants. *Dig Dis Sci*. 2015;60(1):252–259.
14. Calkins KL, Venick RS, and Devaskar SU. Complications associated with parenteral nutrition in the neonate. *Clin Perinatol.* 2014;41:331–345.
15. Zambrano E, El-Hennawy M, Ehrenkranz RA, Zelterman D, Reyes-Mugica M. Total parenteral nutrition induced liver pathology: an autopsy series of 24 cases. *Pediatr Dev Pathol.* 2004;7:425–432.
16. Blackmer AB, Bailey E. Management of copper deficiency in cholestatic infants: Review of the literature and a case series. *Nutr Clin Pract.* 2013;28:75–86.
17. Fok FT, Chui KKM, Cheung R, Ng PC, Cheung CL, Hjelm M. Manganese intake and cholestatic jaundice in neonates receiving parenteral nutrition: a randomized controlled study. *Acta Paediatr.* 2001;90:1009–1015.

18. Chapter 45. Liver disease. In: Kleinman RE and Greer FR, eds. *Pediatric Nutrition, 7th ed.* Elk Grove Village, IL: American Academy of Pediatrics; 2014;1061–1068.
19. Shen YM, Wu JF, Hsu HY, Ni YH, Chang MH, Liu YW, Lai HS, Hsu WM, Weng HL, Chen HL. Oral absorbable fat-soluble vitamin formulation in pediatric patients with cholestasis. *J Pediatr Gastroenterol Nutr.* 2012;55:587–591.
20. Shneider BL, Magee JC, Bezerra JA, Haber B, Karpen SJ, Raghunathan T, Rosenthal P, Schwarz K, Suchy FJ, Kerkar N, Turmelle Y, Whitington PF, Robuck PR, Sokol RJ; Childhood Liver Disease Research Education Network (ChiLDREN). Efficacy of fat-soluble vitamin supplementation in infants with biliary atresia. *Pediatrics.* 2012;130:e607–e614.
21. Westergren T, Kalikstad B. Dosage and formulation issues: oral vitamin E therapy in children. *Eur J Clin Pharmacol.* 2010;66:109–118.
22. Shearer MJ. Vitamin K in Parenteral Nutrition. *Gastroenterol.* 2009;137:S105–S118.
23. Strople J, Lovell G, Heubi J. Prevalence of subclinical vitamin K deficiency in cholestatic liver disease. *J Pediatr Gastroenterol Nutr.* 2009;49:78–84
24. Sokoll LJ, Sadowski JA. Comparison of biochemical indexes for assessing vitamin K nutritional status in a healthy adult population. *Am J Clin Nutr.* 1996;63:566–73.

Chapter 10

Congenital Anomalies of the Alimentary Tract

Amy Jones, MS, RD, LD, CLC

DISEASE STATE

Feeding and nutrition implications deal with three sections of the infant's alimentary tract: (*a*) upper alimentary tract (from mouth through stomach), (*b*) small intestine, and (*c*) large intestine. See Table 10.1 for specific anomalies associated with these sections. Surgical treatment, required for most of these conditions, is followed by a gradual return of alimentary tract function. It is speculated that infants divert protein and energy from growth to tissue repair, thus avoiding the catabolism and hypermetabolism seen in adults. (See Chapter 7, Necrotizing Enterocolitis, and Chapter 8, Short Bowel Syndrome.)

Infants' energy and protein requirements seem to be minimally affected by major surgeries (1). Severity of the metabolic response to injury is reflected in serum C-reactive protein (CRP) levels. When CRP levels are elevated, overfeeding can increase complications and delay recovery (2).

Prealbumin levels are inversely correlated with CRP levels and can be used to gauge return to anabolic metabolism (2,3). Perioperative anesthesia and postoperative analgesia help blunt the metabolic stress response (4).

PREVENTIVE NUTRITION

None.

TREATMENT NUTRITION

The nutrition regimen for infants after alimentary tract surgery (summarized in Table 10.1) includes the following:

- Start parenteral nutrition (PN) soon after surgery. In the acute phase after surgery, while CRP levels are ≥ 2 mg/dL, provide maintenance PN (eg, amino acids 2.5 to 3 g/kg/d, dextrose 8.5 to 10 g/kg/d, and intravenous fat emulsion 1 to 2 g/kg/d) **(B)** (2).
- Encourage mothers to start pumping soon after delivery with a hospital-grade electric breast pump. To establish and maintain a good milk supply, mothers should pump every 2 to 3 hours **(B)** **(C)** (5,6).
- When CRP decreases (indicating reduced metabolic stress) and prealbumin increases (indicating resumption of anabolism), advance nutrient intake as tolerated to promote growth **(B)** (2). After surgical stress, anabolic recovery frequently occurs more rapidly in preterm than in term infants **(B)** (7).
- For infants expected to be on long-term PN, minimize PN-associated cholestasis by avoiding excessive energy (see Chapter 2) **(C)**. Mothers should be encouraged to perform skin-to-skin care and nonnutritive sucking at the breast **(B)** **(C)** (5,6).
- When evidence of intestinal motility returns following surgery, start minimal enteral nutrition (MEN) **(C)**.
- The optimal composition of enteral feedings after alimentary tract surgery is unknown. See options in Table 10.1, which are based on accumulated clinical experience of practitioners **(C)**.

- For preterm infants on protein hydrolysate or amino acid–based formulas, consider a transition to fortified human milk or preterm formula for improved nutritional adequacy **(C)** (8).
- If feeding progression for infants (especially for those with small intestinal anomalies) becomes complicated by significant malabsorption, consider suggestions made earlier for small bowel syndrome.

Table 10.1 Congenital Alimentary Tract Anomalies and Feeding/Nutrition Implications

	Upper Alimentary Tract	Small Intestine	Large Intestine
Specific anomalies	• Cleft lip/cleft palate • Esophageal atresia/ tracheoesophageal fistula • Pyloric stenosis	• Omphalocele • Gastroschisis • Congenital diaphragmatic hernia • Congenital obstruction (atresia, malrotation, and/or volvulus)	• Hirschsprung's disease • Meconium plug • Meconium ileus • Imperforate anus
Feeding/ nutrition challenges	Ingesting and retaining feedings	Digesting and absorbing feedings	Excreting intestinal waste products
Digestion/ absorption affected?	No	Yes	No (unless infant has CF—often associated with meconium ileus)
Long-term PN expected?	No	Yes—provide central venous access early	No

(continued)

Table 10.1 Congenital Alimentary Tract Anomalies and Feeding/Nutrition Implications (continued)

Enteral product(s)	Preterm: human milk (+HMF when 100 mL/kg/d) and/or preterm formula Term: human milk (+direct breastfeeding when tolerated) and/or standard term formula	Preterm and term: human milk, protein hydrolysate, or amino acid–based formulas. Fortification will be needed for preterm infants.	Preterm: human milk (+HMF when 100 mL/kg/d) and/or preterm formula Term: human milk (+direct breastfeeding when tolerated) and/or standard term formula
MEN rate	10–20 mL/kg/d	10–20 mL/kg/d	10–20 mL/kg/d
Progressive feeding rate	≤ 35 mL/kg/d	Individualized; MEN may be maintained for weeks; progressive feedings usually advance slowly (10 mL/kg/d).	≤ 35 mL/kg/d
Feeding methodology	Oral or enteral; infants with cleft lip and/or palate may require feeding evaluation/treatment	Continuous enteral, transition to bolus, if indicated; provide nonnutritive sucking on pacifier.	Oral or enteral
Time to reach full feedings	Rapid: ~1–2 wks	Slow: weeks to months; PN maintained.	Rapid: ~1–2 wks

Abbreviations: CF, cystic fibrosis; PN, parenteral nutrition; HMF: human milk fortifier; MEN, minimal enteral nutrition; NG, nasogastric.
Source: Used by permission of Melody Thompson.

REFERENCES

1. Pierro A, Eaton S. Nutrition in the neonatal surgical patient. In: Thureen PJ, Hay WW Jr, eds. *Neonatal Nutrition and Metabolism.* 2nd ed. New York, NY: Cambridge University Press; 2006:569–585.
2. Alaedeen DI, Queen AL, Leung E, Liu D, Chwals WJ. C-Reactive protein-determined injury severity: length of stay predictor in surgical infants. *J Pediatr Surg.* 2004;39:1832–1834.
3. Ambalavanan N, Ross AC, Carlo WA. Retinol-binding protein, transthyretin, and C-reactive protein in extremely low birth weight (ELBW) infants. *J Perinatol.* 2005;25:714–719.
4. Thureen PJ, Hay WW Jr. Conditions requiring special nutritional management. In: Tsang RC, Uauy R, Koletzko B, Zlotkin SH, eds: *Nutrition of the Preterm Infant: Scientific Basis and Practical Guidelines.* 2nd ed. Cincinnati, OH: Digital Educational Publishing; 2005:393.
5. Spatz DL. Ten steps for promoting and protecting breastfeeding for vulnerable infants. *J Perinat Neonatal Nurs.* 2004;18(4):385–396.
6. Edwards TM, Spatz DL. An innovative model for achieving breast-feeding success in infants with complex surgical anomalies. *J Perinat Neonatal Nurs.* 2010;24(3):246–253.
7. Tueting JL, Byerley LO, Chwals WJ. Anabolic recovery relative to degree of prematurity after acute injury in neonates. *J Pediatr Surg.* 1999;34:13–16.
8. Koo WWK, McLaughlin K, Saba M. Neonatal intensive care. In: Merritt RJ, ed. *The A.S.P.E.N. Nutrition Support Practice Manual.* 2nd ed. Silver Spring, MD: A.S.P.E.N. Publishers; 2005:312.

Chapter 11

Gastroesophageal Reflux Disease

Ann E. Lewis, RD

DISEASE STATE

Gastroesophageal reflux (GER) is the passage of gastric contents into the esophagus with or without regurgitation and vomiting. It is a common physiologic condition in infancy that is benign and self-limiting, typically resolving by 1 year. Incidence is similar in breastfed and formula-fed infants, although duration of episodes may be shorter in breastfed infants (1).

Gastroesophageal reflux disease (GERD) is reflux that is accompanied by esophageal or extraesophageal-related pathology (2). Esophageal symptoms can include dysphagia, vomiting, esophagitis, and abdominal pain; extraesophageal conditions manifest as respiratory disorders (cough, laryngitis, and wheezing); or poor weight gain. GERD frequently manifests in neurodevelopmental disabilities and some surgical alimentary tract anomalies (1–5).

A dual 24-hour pH probe and multiple intraluminal impedance, an emerging diagnostic modality study, are recommended to diagnose GERD and to temporally relate particular symptoms (eg, apnea, cough, and other respiratory and behavioral symptoms) **(C)** (1). Routine testing of gastric emptying via nuclear scintigraphy is not recommended to diagnose GERD, but has value when symptoms of gastric retention are present (1). An upper gastrointestinal (UGI) series is neither sensitive nor specific in diagnosing GERD, but is useful in detecting anatomical abnormalities (eg, transesophageal fistula or pyloric stenosis) **(B)** (1).

PREVENTIVE NUTRITION

Currently, there are no strategies to prevent GERD, only treatment modalities to minimize the associated symptoms.

TREATMENT NUTRITION

Parental education and reassurance are the primary interventions indicated for GER **(C)**. Current evidence does not support other interventions (1). The following nutrition interventions have shown some efficacy in infantile GERD. The treatment options are in recommended order of initiation:

- Small, frequent (or continuous) feedings are associated with fewer episodes of GER than are larger, less frequent feedings **(B,C)** (1,3). Transpyloric tube feedings, when compared with gastric tube feedings, were found to increase GI disturbances and mortality in preterm infants without an identified benefit **(A)** (6).
- Prone and left lateral positioning have been associated with less reflux (1,4,7). Since delayed gastric emptying is observed to a greater degree in infant reflux, one study recommended placing the infant in a right lateral position for the first hour to promote

gastric emptying, followed by a left lateral position to decrease reflux **(C)** (8). At home, due to sudden infant death syndrome concerns, infants should lie supine when sleeping and supine or prone after feedings or when the infant is awake **(A)** (4,7). In some infants, a cow's milk protein allergy or other formula intolerance can cause symptoms (eg, irritability, distress, and vomiting) that are indistinguishable from GERD and can be successfully treated by hypoallergenic feedings (90% of infants will not have a reaction) or nonallergenic feedings (100% of infants will not have a reaction) (4,5). Changing from a cow's milk–based formula to an amino acid–based or casein hydrolysate formula decreases spitting up/vomiting in as many as half of formula-fed infants with GERD. A 1- to 2-week trial of a hypoallergenic formula is recommended; continue if efficacy is seen **(A)** (5,9). These products are formulated with nutrient levels for full-term infants; if used for more than 1 week in preterm infants, assess adequacy of nutrient intake. Nutrient supplementation, particularly minerals, is often indicated **(C)**. If allergy is suspected in a breastfed infant, the lactating mother should initiate a 2- to 4-week trial eliminating cow's milk and eggs. If the infant's condition does not improve, her dietary restrictions should be discontinued **(C)**.

- Thickened feedings
  - Thickened feedings reduce regurgitation (symptomatic reflux), but do not reduce the reflux index (the amount of time that the esophagus is bathed in acidic fluid) and may also increase coughing **(A)** (4,7). Thickened feedings are not possible or desirable with direct breastfeeding. Pumped, fresh breastmilk cannot be thickened with cereal or

starches (presumably due to the amylase activity in the milk) **(C)**.

- Carob thickeners have been associated with diarrhea and allergic reaction (9). Studies reporting the safety of using locust bean gum (also called carob bean gum) to thicken feedings only include term infants less than 12 weeks of age with uncomplicated GER **(C)** (10).
- Caution has also been advised when using xanthan gum–based or similar thickening agents in infants born with anomalies including abdominal wall and congenital heart defects (11). The US Food and Drug Administration (FDA) issued a warning in 2011 that "parents, caregivers and health care providers not . . . feed 'Simply Thick®' to infants born before 37 weeks' gestation who are currently receiving hospital care or have been discharged from the hospital in the past 30 days" due to its possible association with necrotizing enterocolitis (NEC) (2). This advisory warning was expanded to term infants in 2012 (11).
- In neonatal intensive care units (NICUs) in the United States, formulas have traditionally been thickened with dry infant rice cereal. Concerns about the safety of dried or powdered products in the NICU may preclude the use of dry cereal or other powdered thickeners (12). Adding cereal to feedings may also provide excess calories as carbohydrate, since 1 tablespoon of rice cereal added to a 20 kcal/oz formula increases the caloric density to 34 kcal/oz (2).
- US and European studies on commercial infant formulas that contain part of their carbohydrate as rice starch, which thickens at gastric pH, have

been shown to decrease the amount and severity of regurgitation **(A)** (4,5,14). However, concomitant use of acid-suppressant medications likely diminishes the efficacy of these formulas **(C)**. In vitro studies have shown decreased availability of minerals and micronutrients in commercially thickened formulas that contain indigestible, but not digestible, fiber **(B)** (1). The nutrient profiles of these formulas are intended for term infants. The risks and benefits should be considered in the context of prescribing these for preterm or former preterm infants, with individual nutrients added as needed **(C)**.

ADDITIONAL TREATMENT OPTIONS

Medication

Acid-suppressant and prokinetic medications may be beneficial **(A,B,C)** (4,7). Histamine-2 receptor antagonists (H2RA) alleviate reflux symptoms and promote healing. Proton pump inhibitors (PPIs) are superior to H2RAs in relief of both GERD symptoms and esophagitis **(A)**. However, studies suggest that acid suppressants and prokinetic agents with either H2RAs or PPIs increase the risk for developing community-acquired pneumonia, gastroenteritis, candidemia, and NEC in preterm infants **(B)** (2).

Surgery

Surgical fundoplication may be indicated for severe cases **(C)** (13).

REFERENCES

1. Vandenplas Y, Rudolph CD, Di Lorenzo C, Hassall E, Liptak G, Mazur L, Sondheimer J, Staiano A, Thomson M, Veereman-Wauters G, Wenzl TG; North American Society for Pediatric Gastroenterology Hepatology and Nutrition, European Society for Pediatric Gastroenterology Hepatology and Nutrition. Pediatric gastroesophageal reflux clinical practice guidelines: joint recommendations of the North American Society for Pediatric Gastroenterology, Hepatology and Nutrition (NASPGHAN) and the European Society for Pediatric Gastroenterology, Hepatology and Nutrition (ESPGHAN). *J Pediatr Gastroenterol Nutr.* 2009;49:498–547.
2. Lightdale JR, Gremse DA Section on Gastroenterology, Hepatology, and Nutrition. Gastroesophageal reflux: management guidance for the pediatrician. *Pediatrics.* 2013;131(5):e1684–e1695.
3. Thompson M. Gastroesophageal reflux. In: Groh-Wargo S, Thompson M, Cox JH, eds. *Nutritional Care for High-Risk Newborns.* 3rd ed. Chicago, IL: Precept Press; 2000:460–461.
4. Rudolph CD, Mazur LJ, Liptak GS, Baker RD, Boyle JT, Colletti RB, Gerson WT, Werlin SL; North American Society for Pediatric Gastroenterology and Nutrition. Guidelines for evaluation and treatment of gastroesophageal reflux in infants and children: recommendations of the North American Society for Pediatric Gastroenterology and Nutrition. *J Pediatr Gastroenterol Nutr.* 2001;32(Suppl 2):S1–S31.
5. Salvatore S, Vandenplas Y. Gastroesophageal reflux and cow milk allergy: is there a link? *Pediatrics.* 2002;110:972–984.
6. Watson J, McGuire W. Transpyloric versus gastric tube feeding for preterm infants. *Cochrane Database Syst Rev.* 2013;(2):CD003487. doi: 10.1002/14651858.CD003487.pub3
7. Craig WR, Hanlon-Dearman A, Sinclair C, Taback S, Moffatt M. Metaclopramide, thickened feedings, and positioning for gastroesophageal reflux in children under two years. *Cochrane Database Syst Rev.* 2004;(4):CD003502.
8. van Wijk MP, Benninga MA, Dent J, Lontis R, Goodchild L, McCall LM, Haslam R, Davidson GP, Omari T. Effect of body position changes on postprandial gastroesophageal reflux and gastric emptying in the healthy premature neonate. *J Pediatr.* 2007;151:585–590.

9. Horvath A, Dziechciarz P, Szajewska H. The effect of thickened-feed interventions on gastroesophageal reflux in infants: systematic review and meta-analysis of randomized, controlled trials. *Pediatrics.* 2008;122(6):e1268–e1276.
10. Meunier L, Garthoff JA, Schaafsma A, Krul L, Schrijver J, van Goudoever JB, Speijers G, Vandenplas Y. Locust bean gum safety in neonates and young infants: an integrated review of the toxicological database and clinical evidence. *Regul Toxicol Pharmacol.* 2014;70(6):155–169.
11. American Academy of Pediatrics. Thickening agent caution expanded to term infants. *AAP News*. Sept 19, 2012. doi: 10.1542/aapnews.20120919-1. http://aapnews.aappublications.org/content/early/2012/09/19/aapnews.20120919-1. Accessed May 5, 2015.
12. Lin LC, Beuchat LR. Survival of *Enterobacter sakazakii* in infant cereal as affected by composition, water activity, and temperature. *Food Microbiol.* 2007;24:767–777.
13. Pacilli M, Chowdhury MM, Pierro A. The surgical treatment of gastro-esophageal reflux in neonates and infants. *Semin Pediatr Surg.* 2005;14:34–41.
14. Lasekan JB, Hawley KL, Oliver JS, Carver JD, Blatter MM, Kuchan MJ, Cramer JM, Pollack PF. Milk protein-based infant formula containing rice starch and low lactose reduces common regurgitation in healthy term infants: a randomized, blinded and prospective trial. *J Am Coll Nutr.* 2014:33(2);136–146.

Chapter 12

Renal Function

Allison Prince, MS, RDN, LD

DISEASE STATE (1–4)

Causes of Dysfunction

Renal function may be compromised during the neonatal period due to:

- Prerenal clinical conditions that may cause decreased renal perfusion: dehydration, excessive gastrointestinal (GI) fluid loss, blood loss, perinatal asphyxia, hypotension, sepsis, or patent ductus arteriosus
- Intrinsic renal disease: acute tubular necrosis or congenital abnormalities
- Postrenal obstructions: congenital anomalies or fungal infections within the urinary tract
- Functional renal immaturity in preterm infants, which increases risk for dehydration, hyponatremia, metabolic acidosis, mild azotemia, hyperkalemia, and increased losses of glucose, zinc, and some water-soluble vitamins
- Nephrocalcinosis, which is more common in preterm infants due to immature renal function, hypercalciuria, low glomerular filtration rate, low citrate excretion, alkaline urine, excessive vitamin D intake, phosphorus depletion, and acid/base imbalances, but resolves over time

Assessment of Renal Function

Prerenal failure, or decreased renal perfusion, may be differentiated from intrinsic renal disease by measuring fractional sodium excretion or by the renal failure index (3):

$$RFI = \frac{U_{Na} \times P_{Cr}}{U_{Cr}}$$

Where: RFI is renal failure index, U_{Na} refers to urine sodium in mg/dL, P_{Cr} refers to plasma creatinine in mg/dL, and U_{Cr} refers to urine creatinine in mg/dL. An RFI $>$ 8 indicates intrinsic renal disease. Improvement of urine output following a 10 mL/kg isotonic saline bolus confirms prerenal causes for abnormal lab values that are used to measure renal function.

Acute kidney injury (AKI), which is the preferred term to renal insufficiency, is characterized by urine output $<$ 0.5 mL/kg/h; elevations of serum creatinine, potassium, and phosphorus levels; edema; and altered electrolyte and acid/base balance (5). Nonoliguric AKI is characterized by an increase in serum creatinine. To calculate creatinine clearance (1):

$$CrCl\ (mL/min/1.73\ m^2) = \frac{K \times Length\ (cm)}{P_{Cr}}$$

Where: CrCl is creatinine clearance; K is a constant = 0.34 in preterm infants up to 34 weeks' gestational age (GA); K= 0.44 in infants 35 weeks' GA to term; and P_{Cr} = plasma creatinine in mg/dL.

Plasma creatinine of 1.5 mg/dL (or 132.5 micromol/L) for $>$ 24 hours, consistent with a 50% reduction in creatinine clearance, is often used to define AKI.

Chronic kidney disease (CKD) includes the same biochemical changes that occur in AKI, but may also include anemia, renal osteodystrophy, anorexia, and poor growth.

PREVENTIVE NUTRITION (1–4, 6–7)

In prerenal causes of renal failure, provide adequate fluid and electrolytes to maintain normal hydration and electrolyte and acid/base status **(C)**.

In cases of nephrocalcinosis, the following is advised:

- Maintain acid/base balance; prevent hypophosphatemia **(C)**.
- Ensure adequate fluid, protein, and energy intake when providing increased amounts of calcium and phosphorus to support intrauterine rates of linear growth **(C)**.
- Vitamin D: doses of 200 to 400 IU/d are adequate **(C)**.
- Consider assessment of urine calcium-to-creatinine ratio in infants who require chronic diuretic or steroid medications, when mineral supplements are given to treat osteopenia, or when vitamin D is given in doses > 400 IU/d. Urine calcium-to-creatinine ratios > 1.5 mmol calcium/mmol creatinine may indicate excessive calcium excretion and increased risk of nephrocalcinosis **(B)** (8).

TREATMENT NUTRITION (1–7, 9–12)

Fluid and Electrolytes

- In oliguria and anuria, fluid intake = urine output + insensible losses (generally 25 to 30 mL/kg/d for most infants, but may be higher for infants who are < 26 weeks' GA). As fluids may be restricted to < 100 mL/kg/d, considerable effort may be needed to provide adequate amounts of nutrients.
- Sodium (1 to 3 mEq/kg/d) and potassium (1 to 2 mEq/kg/d) intake may need to be restricted. Bicarbonate

supplementation of 1 to 2 mEq/kg/d may be needed to achieve acid/base balance and prevent hyperkalemia. Restrict potassium intake by limiting or removing potassium in intravenous fluids and enteral feeds. Treatment of formula or human milk with an ion exchange resin, such as sodium polysteryne sulfonate (SPS), reduces the potassium content of the feeding. Human milk or formula should then be decanted so that it can be fed to the infant (9).

- In high-output renal failure, fluid needs may be 150 to 200 mL/kg/d. Supplements of sodium and/or bicarbonate of 5 to 10 mEq/kg/d may be needed.
- In urinary, stool, or dialysate losses, replace fluids and electrolytes as needed to maintain homeostasis.

Energy

Calculation of energy needs should be individualized to promote normal growth/anabolism and to prevent catabolism. For premature infants, 120 kcal/kg/d is often prescribed; otherwise, 100% of the Estimated Energy Requirement (EER) is recommended for infants 0–12 months and adjusted as needed based on weight loss/gain (7,10).

Peritoneal dialysate solutions provide substantial amounts of energy as dextrose and must be included when assessing energy intake. Energy intake needs to be adjusted individually because absorbed dextrose depends on dwell time, dextrose concentration, and individual absorption gradient.

Anorexia associated with azotemia and limited fluid intake may require use of a nutrient-dense formula, modular additives, and/or supplemental tube feedings (see Chapter 3, Enteral Nutrition). Carbohydrate or fat modular additives may be added to human milk or infant formulas to achieve adequate intake and growth, especially if protein, phosphorus, and/or potassium intake must be restricted (see Chapter 3, Enteral Nutrition).

Increase energy density of feedings gradually to help promote tolerance. Additional carbohydrate (35% to 65% of total energy) and/or fat (30% to 55% of total energy) may be needed to meet energy needs (meet protein, mineral, and vitamin needs before adding modular sources of additional energy).

Protein

There are no studies that have identified specific protein requirements in the preterm infant with AKI or CKD. Protein needs have been estimated at 1.5 to 2.5 g/kg/d in the preterm infant with AKI (10). Term infants ages 0 to 6 months with CKD require 1.5 to 2.1 g/kg/d or 100% to 140% of the Dietary Reference Intake (DRI) for ideal body weight. For infants ages 7 to 12 months, protein needs are 1.2 to 1.7 g/kg/d. Maximum protein needs decrease as the stage of CKD progresses without renal replacement therapy **(C)** (7).

For peritoneal dialysis, protein needs may be more than the DRI for age, or 1.5 to 1.8 g/kg/d in term infants and ranging from 4 to 6 g/kg/d in premature infants **(C)** (7,11). For hemodialysis, protein needs are 1.6 g/kg/d for infants ages 0 to 6 months and 1.3 g/kg/d for infants ages 7 to 12 months. These amounts are lower than previous recommendations, reflecting changes in the DRIs.

Calcium

In CKD, calcium needs are 210 to 420 mg/d for ages 0 to 6 months and 270 to 540 mg/d for ages 7 to 12 months **(C)** (7).

In hypocalcemia, dihydrotachysterol (DHT) or calcitriol forms of vitamin D and additional calcium supplements as calcium carbonate liquid suspension in doses of 0.2 to 0.8 mL/kg/d may be needed (250 mg calcium carbonate or 100 mg elemental calcium per 1 mL).

In nephrocalcinosis, provide the DRI or recommended intake for age for phosphorus, fluid, protein, energy. Avoid excessive vitamin D intake.

Phosphorus

Infants, particularly preterm infants, are rapidly growing and mineralizing bone tissue. If at the same time, renal excretion of excess phosphorus is decreased, it is important to provide up to but not greater than standard amounts of phosphorus as long as serum levels are within the normal range. While specific recommendations for preterm infants are lacking, phosphorus intake for term infants should be limited to ≤ 100% of the DRI. Phosphorus intakes for infants ages 0 to 6 months should be ≤ 100 mg/d, and for infants 7 to 12 months, ≤ 275 mg/d **(C)** (7).

Serum phosphorus levels should be carefully reviewed, as the normal range for serum phosphorus varies by age. If hyperphosphatemia is present, decrease phosphorus by 30% to 50% when parenteral nutrition (PN) is provided. For EN or oral feedings, a formula with lower phosphorus content or human milk may be needed to support normal phosphorus levels. To maintain serum phosphorus levels within the normal range, calcium carbonate may be given as a phosphorus binder to increase phosphorus excretion, and doses can be adjusted as needed.

For hypophosphatemia, use standard infant formula; supplement human milk with human milk fortifier for preterm infants, adjusting the amount of fortification as needed to support normal serum phosphorus levels. For term infants, supplement human milk with standard infant formula or sodium phosphate.

Iron

Standard iron doses of 2 to 6 mg/kg/d (based on the individual infant's iron status) are recommended.

Trace minerals (12)

- Zinc: High-output renal failure may require up to 600 mcg/kg/d parenterally. Dialysis, both hemodialysis and peritoneal dialysis, may incur increased losses and require supplementation.
- Chromium, molybdenum, and selenium: Normal excretion may be decreased in renal failure; decrease or omit from parenteral solutions if creatinine > 1 mg/dL.

Aluminum

Infants with compromised renal function are at greater risk of aluminum retention and development of neurotoxicity. When treating hypocalcemia, avoid calcium gluconate due to its higher aluminum content. Aluminum hydroxide binders should also be avoided in the management of hyperphosphatemia. Soy-based formulas have comparatively high amounts of aluminum and are not recommended for infants with reduced renal function (13).

Vitamins

A standard dose of infant liquid multivitamins is recommended, or a small dose of an adult renal multivitamin can be given enterally to meet requirements in infants undergoing dialysis. Ensure folic acid needs are met (1 mg/d) (10).

REFERENCES

1. Edelmann CM, ed. *Pediatric Kidney Disease.* 2nd ed. Boston, MA: Little, Brown, and Co; 1992.

2. Moghal NE, Embleton ND. Management of acute renal failure in the newborn. *Semin Fetal Neonatal Med.* 2006;11:207–213.
3. Haycock GB. Management of acute and chronic renal failure in the newborn. *Semin Neonatol.* 2003;8:325–334.
4. Hein G, Richter D, Manz F, Weitzel D, Kalhoff H. Development of nephrocalcinosis in very low birth weight infants. *Pediatr Nephrol.* 2004;19:616–620.
5. Jetton JG, Askenazi DJ. Acute Kidney Injury in the Neonate. *Clin Perinatol.* 2014; 41:487–502.
6. Spinozzi N. Renal dysfunction. In: Groh-Wargo S, Thompson M, Cox JH, eds. *Nutritional Care for High-Risk Newborns.* 3rd ed. Chicago, IL: Precept Press; 2000:507–520.
7. National Kidney Foundation. KDOQI Clinical Practice Guideline for Nutrition in Children with CKD: 2008 Update. *Am J Kidney Dis.* 2009;53:S1–S124.
8. Metz MP. Determining urinary calcium/creatinine cut-offs for paediatric population using published data. *Ann Clin Biochem.* 2006;43:398–401.
9. Thompson K, Flynn J, Okamura D, Zhou L. Pretreatment of formula or expressed breast milk with sodium polystyrene sulfonate (Kayexalate®) as a treatment for hyperkalemia in infants with acute or chronic renal insufficiency. *J Ren Nutr.* 2013;23(5):333–339.
10. Corkins MR, ed. *The A.S.P.E.N. Pediatric Nutrition Support Core Curriculum.* Silver Spring, MD: American Society for Parenteral and Enteral Nutrition; 2010:256–282.
11. Rainey KE, DiGeronimo RJ, Pascual-Baralt J. Successful long-term peritoneal dialysis in a very low birth weight infant with renal failure secondary to feto-fetal transfusion syndrome. *Pediatrics.* 2000;106:849–851.
12. Greene H, Hambidge K, Schanler R, Tsang RC. Guidelines for the use of vitamins, trace elements, calcium, magnesium, and phosphorus in infants and children receiving total parenteral nutrition: report of the Subcommittee on Pediatric Parenteral Nutrient Requirements from the Committee on Clinical Practice Issues of the American Society for Clinical Nutrition. *Am J Clin Nutr.* 1988;48:1324–1342.
13. Bhatia J, Greer F, Committee on Nutrition. Use of soy protein-based formulas in infant feeding. *Pediatrics.* 2008;121:1062–1068.

Chapter 13

Neurology and Metabolic Disorders

Hunter Rametta, MS, RDN, LDN, CNSC

DISEASE STATE

Neurologic impairment may be caused by the following (1):

- Genetic factors: chromosomal abnormalities, inherited neurometabolic disorders (inborn errors of metabolism), or neuromuscular disorders
- Congenital disorders/birth defects: drug exposure, fetal alcohol syndrome, hydrocephalus, spina bifida, intrauterine growth retardation, intrauterine infections, uncontrolled maternal neurometabolic conditions during pregnancy
- Perinatal trauma: asphyxia (hypoxic ischemic encephalopathy), intraventricular hemorrhage, meconium aspiration, or septic shock

PREVENTIVE NUTRITION

Specific nutrition-related strategies to prevent neurologic diseases are generally not known, other than the following **(B)** (1–4):

- Spina bifida has a genetic etiology, but considerable evidence suggests that adequate maternal intake of folic acid (400 mcg/d) throughout childbearing years and pregnancies can significantly reduce risk.
- Dietary treatment of neurometabolic disorders during pregnancy is generally recommended to reduce risk of neurologic compromise in the infant.
- Abstinence from alcohol throughout pregnancy is recommended to prevent fetal alcohol syndrome.

TREATMENT NUTRITION

Many neurometabolic disorders are amenable to nutrition therapy, but nutrition treatment modalities for infants with other neurological conditions relate primarily to problems of altered growth and energy needs, abnormal muscle tone, delayed feeding skills, dysphagia, gastroesophageal reflux, constipation, and/or drug-nutrient interactions (1–4).

Infants may require several complex nutrition strategies to provide treatment and prevent neurological dysfunction. Specific nutrition treatment strategies are beyond the scope of this pocket guide (see references 2 and 3), but generally fall into one or more of the following categories **(B)** (1–4):

- Prevent catabolism by avoiding fasting and providing adequate energy to meet metabolic demands for normal growth and development, especially during periods of illness or stress when oral intake may be limited.
- Restrict dietary intake of specific nutrient(s) to prevent toxic accumulation due to lack of enzymes or blocked/impaired metabolic pathways.
- Supplement nutrients that help drive alternate metabolic pathways, become essential due to lack of

endogenous production or blocked metabolic pathways, replace deficient cofactors or induce normal enzyme production, and are inadequately absorbed or not available metabolically.

Growth Assessment

Growth may be altered in infants with neurologic compromise **(C)**. Head circumference may be disproportional to length and weight on growth charts. Normal head-to-length proportion is described by the following equation (5):

$$\text{Head circumference (cm)} = (0.5\ \text{length [cm]} + 9.5) \pm 2.5\ \text{cm}$$

Anthropometric assessment should be done using World Health Organization (WHO)/Centers for Disease Control (CDC) growth charts for all infants once beyond term-corrected age. Specialized growth charts exist for children with a variety of disabilities. However, it is important to note that these are descriptive growth charts showing *how* these populations grow. They are not intended to be prescriptive, describing how they *should* grow (4,6). Infants with intrauterine growth restriction associated with drug or alcohol exposure, intrauterine infection, or microcephaly may not experience catch-up growth.

Energy

Although not specifically predictable, variations in energy needs may be expected **(C)** (4,6). Resting metabolic rate may be lower, decreasing energy needs if brain tissue mass or function is below normal.

Energy needs may be increased to accommodate increased muscle tone, seizure activity, irritability, or spasticity/involuntary movement. Energy needs may be decreased when muscle tone or movement is below normal. Energy needs for growth may be decreased for specific diagnoses and syndromes associated with decreased growth potential.

When energy needs are less than 75 kcal/kg/d, protein, electrolyte, vitamin, and mineral supplements may be required to meet Dietary Reference Intakes (DRIs).

Delayed Feeding Skills/Dysphagia **(C)**

Hunger/satiety cues may be subtle or absent in infants with neurologic disorders, and caregiver(s) may need help interpreting cues. If oral feedings take longer than 20 to 30 minutes, consider supplemental tube feedings to prevent fatigue and feeding aversion (1). If calorie-dense formula is used to provide adequate nutrition in a tolerated volume, ensure that adequate fluid intake (minimum of 100 mL/kg/d free water) is provided. Educate caregiver(s) about the signs and symptoms of dehydration.

Tube feeding recommendations include the following (6,7):

- For short-term (< 2 months) tube feeding, use a nasogastric feeding tube. An orogastric feeding tube may be needed to prevent airway obstruction in a younger infant, but this may also interfere with oral skill development. Either type of tube may stimulate the gag reflex and contribute to feeding aversion. Feeding therapy should be started to promote and develop oral skills and to minimize feeding aversion.
- For long-term (> 2 months) tube feeding, a gastrostomy tube is recommended because it is safer for continuous feedings and diminishes noxious facial stimulation associated with nasogastric or orogastric feeding tubes. Gastrostomy feedings may increase

gastroesophageal reflux (GER). Including oral therapy at feeding times is recommended as it may improve feeding skills.

- For infants with absent gag reflex or recurrent pneumonia, a jejunal tube may be needed.

If tube feedings are required at the time of discharge (1), consider the following:

- Provide caregiver(s) with expected weight gain and volume progression to support normal weight gain until nutrition follow-up can be scheduled.
- Ensure adequacy of intake for all nutrients, including fluid and electrolytes.
- Educate caregiver(s) to use hunger and satiety cues as much as possible to facilitate eventual oral feeding; do not force feed.
- Provide caregiver(s) with guidelines to make feedings as normal as possible: holding infant, pleasant facial stimulation, social interaction, temperature of feeding, duration of feeding, etc.
- Collaboration with an interdisciplinary team is crucial to individualize a feeding plan to best meet the needs of both the infant and caregiver(s). Some infants may be able to nipple part of each feeding, or several feedings each day with supplemental tube feeding given simultaneously with oral feeding, as a bolus after the oral feeding, or as a continuous feeding at night.
- For oral-motor skill development, indwelling nasogastric tubes are generally preferred over orogastric tubes, but either may be used if tube feedings will be required for a short period (up to 2 to 3 months). If tube feedings are required for longer periods of time, gastrostomy feeding tube placement is generally recommended to reduce risk of oral aversion.

If thickened liquids are needed to facilitate swallowing:

- Ensure feeding recommendations meet all nutrient needs without providing excessive energy; instruct caregiver(s) about accurate preparation of feedings.
- Rice starch–containing formulas that are used for GER have a higher viscosity than standard formulas and may be of nearly nectar consistency without providing excessive carbohydrate intake. Of note, these formulas thicken upon contact with an acidic environment. Therefore, infants on acid-blocking therapy would not benefit from these formulas. (See Chapter 3, Enteral Nutrition.)
- Starch-based thickeners are quickly inactivated by breast milk amylase. See Chapter 11, Gastroesophageal Reflux Disease, for a more thorough discussion on thickeners.

Gastroesophageal Reflux

See Chapter 11, Gastroesophageal Reflux Disease.

Constipation

Constipation is often associated with decreased bowel motility, alterations in abdominal muscle tone, decreased activity, low fluid intake, frequent vomiting, and/or medications (4) **(C)**.

- Ensure adequate fluid intake—free water of at least 100 mL/kg/d. Additional water may be needed to replace increased losses.
- Avoid chronic use of laxatives or enemas to prevent dependency and/or nutrient loss, particularly vitamins A, D, E, and K with use of mineral oil.
- Provide 1 to 2 tsp (5 to 10 mL) of prune juice/day or 1 to 2 oz (30 to 60 mL) of pear or apple juice per day if infant is beyond term age.

- Consult an occupational or physical therapist for abdominal massage techniques and range-of-motion exercises for lower extremities.

Drug-Nutrient Interactions

Drugs commonly used in the treatment of neurologically compromised infants include anticonvulsants, antibiotics, drugs that reduce gastric acid or enhance gastric motility, stool softeners, and laxatives (4,6). Antiepileptic drugs, such as phenytoin and phenobarbital, may affect vitamin D metabolism (6). Ensuring adequate vitamin D intake and regular monitoring of 25(OH)D levels approximately every 6 months is recommended.

REFERENCES

1. Nevin-Folino NL. Neurological impairment. In: Groh-Wargo S, Thompson M, Cox JH, eds. *Nutritional Care for High-Risk Newborns*. 3rd ed. Chicago, IL: Precept Press; 2000: 521–534.
2. Acosta P, ed. *Nutrition Management of Patients with Inherited Metabolic Disorders*. Sudbury, MA: Jones and Bartlett; 2010.
3. Acosta P. Genetic Screening and Nutrition Management. In: Samour PQ, King K, eds. *Pediatric Nutrition*. 4th ed. Boston, MA: Jones and Bartlett; 2012:179–217.
4. Cloud HH. Developmental disabilities. In: Samour PQ, King K, eds. *Pediatric Nutrition*. 4th ed. Boston, MA: Jones and Bartlett; 2012:219–238.
5. Dine MS, Gartside PS, Glueck CJ, Rheins L, Greene G, Khoury P. Relationship of head circumference to length in the first 400 days of life: A Mnemonic. *Pediatrics*. 1981;67:506–507.
6. American Academy of Pediatrics Committee on Nutrition. Nutritional support for children with developmental disabilities. In: Kleinman RE, Greer FR, eds. *Pediatric Nutrition*. 7th ed. Elk Grove Village, IL: American Academy of Pediatrics; 2014: 883–899.
7. Wessel JJ. Feeding methodologies. In: Groh-Wargo S, Thompson M, Cox JH, eds. *Nutritional Care for High Risk Newborns*. 3rd ed. Chicago, IL: Precept Press; 2000: 341–355.

Chapter 14

Endocrinology

Amy Gates, RD, CSP, LD

DISEASE STATE

Endocrine disorders requiring nutritional management generally involve glucose or calcium metabolism. Deficiencies in thyroid, growth, or pituitary hormone often present with poor feeding and poor growth. Hormone replacement therapy obviates dietary management beyond monitoring feeding progression and growth recovery (1–3).

Hypoglycemia

Although controversy exists regarding screening guidelines and the specific glucose levels that define hypoglycemia, the American Academy of Pediatrics has defined hypoglycemia as plasma glucose levels < 45 mg/dL (2.5 mMol/L) when accompanied by signs or symptoms of hypoglycemia (eg, for example, irritability, tremors, jitteriness, lethargy, low muscle tone, cyanosis, apnea, etc.) or levels < 36 mg/dL (2.0 mMol/L) without symptoms, but accompanied by risk factors (4–6). These risk factors may include (6):

- Endocrine disorders: hyperinsulinism (transient: infant of diabetic mothers, Beckwith-Wiedemann syndrome, asphyxia, and intrauterine growth restriction; persistent: nesidioblastosis, islet cell adenoma);

cortisol or growth hormone deficiencies; panhypopituitarism; hypothyroidism
- Sepsis, polycythemia
- Inborn errors of carbohydrate metabolism: galactosemia, glycogen storage disease, fructose intolerance, glucose-6-phosphate deficiency
- Disorders of fatty acid oxidation: medium chain acyl-CoA or other fatty acid dehydrogenase deficiency; carnitine deficiency (characterized by decreased production of ketones)
- Amino acid disorders: maple syrup urine disease, proprionic acidemia, methylmalonic acidemia and hereditary tyrosinemia
- Iatrogenic causes: hypothermia, delayed feeding, abruptly discontinuing glucose infusions, exchange transfusions

Hyperglycemia

Hyperglycemia is most often encountered in extremely low birth weight (ELBW) infants receiving parenteral nutrition (PN) and is thought to be related to inefficient insulin secretory ability and relative tissue insensitivity to insulin. There is controversy regarding the specific serum glucose level that defines hyperglycemia: definitions include > 144 mg/dL (> 8 mM/L), > 158 mg/dL (> 8.8 mM/L), > 178 mg/L (> 10 mM/L), > 216 mg/dL (>12 mM/L), or > 239 mg/dL (> 13.3 mM/L) (7). Severe hyperglycemia ≥ 180 mg/dL (≥ 10 mM/L) or prolonged hyperglycemia >150 mg/dL (8.3 mM/L) during the first week of life may be associated with increased risk of death or late onset sepsis, dehydration, and electrolyte losses (7,8).

Transient neonatal diabetes mellitus may present in the first 6 weeks of life, usually resolving by 3 to 6 months of age. Neonatal onset of permanent diabetes mellitus may be caused by pancreatic agenesis or other rare congenital disorders.

Hypocalcemia

Early hypocalcemia results from declining serum calcium levels after birth, reflecting the infant's loss of maternal source of calcium, and may be exacerbated by prematurity, asphyxia, sepsis, intrauterine growth restriction, or maternal diabetes and may progress to pathologic hypocalcemia. Symptoms of hypocalcemia include high-pitched cry, jitteriness, and seizures. Endocrine-related causes include hypoparathyroidism, either transient (as in premature infants) or permanent (as in DiGeorge syndrome), pseudohypoparathyroidism, or maternal vitamin D deficiency (1,2).

Hypercalcemia

Endocrine causes of hypercalcemia include primary neonatal hyperparathyroidism or William's Syndrome (2).

PREVENTIVE NUTRITION

Hypoglycemia

Use a screening protocol to identify hypoglycemia, particularly for infants at increased risk **(B)** (4,6).

If medically stable and feedings may be given, provide 10 mL/kg/feeding of human milk or infant formula. Encourage enteral/oral feeding within the first 6 hours of life, or within the first 30 to 60 minutes of life for infants at higher risk for developing hypoglycemia. If feedings are precluded by a medical condition, initiate intravenous dextrose at 4 to 6 mg/kg/min (normal rate of hepatic production of glucose) for term infants, although preterm infants or infants with symmetrical growth restriction may require up to 6 to 8 mg/kg/min to support euglycemia **(C)** (9).

Hyperglycemia

Amino acid administration within the first hours of life may help stimulate endogenous production and secretion of insulin, reducing the need for insulin infusion, particularly in ELBW infants, whose endogenous protein stores are low **(B)**. Parenteral glucose infusion rates greater than 10–11 mg/kg/min may increase the risk for hyperglycemia (10).

TREATMENT NUTRITION

Hypoglycemia

If hypoglycemia is present, but the infant is asymptomatic, start feedings within 1 hour and continue to offer feedings every 2 to 3 hours. If hypoglycemia persists or infant becomes symptomatic, recommendations are generally as follows (1,5,6,11):

- Initiate intravenous glucose infusion to provide 4 to 6 mg/kg/min.
- If plasma glucose is less than 36 mg/dL (2 mMol/L), provide glucose infusion of 6 to 8 mg/kg/min.
- If plasma glucose is less than 25 mg/dL (1.4 mMol/L), provide a bolus of 200 to 250 mg/kg as 10% dextrose over 2 to 5 minutes, then continuous glucose infusion rate (GIR) of 6 to 8 mg/kg/min.
- Increase GIR by 10% to 15% until serum glucose is within normal range.

- If the GIR required to maintain euglycemia exceeds 12 to 15 mg/kg/min, consider medical treatment with glucagon, diazoxide, or octreotide **(C)** (1,5,6).

Infants of mothers with diabetes may present with hypoglycemia, but also with hypocalcemia, hypomagnesemia, and macrosomia. Some may exhibit hypotonia and poor nippled intake due to immature feeding skills **(C)** (12,13). Recommendations for these infants include the following (6,11):

- Give parenteral or enteral calcium and magnesium to correct serum levels if needed.
- Monitor infant's ability to nipple adequate fluid and energy intake to maintain normal hydration and euglycemia, supplementing intake enterally as needed.
- Because infants of mothers with diabetes may exhibit immature feeding skills, they may not achieve standard nippled intakes for actual weight during the first 2 weeks of life. If birth weight is above the 90th percentile, using actual weight to estimate energy requirements may result in overfeeding. Although weight-for-length charts may be used to estimate energy needs based on ideal weight rather than actual weight, intake must also maintain normal hydration and euglycemia.
- To ensure adequate fluid and carbohydrate intake after discharge, provide guidelines for caregiver(s) if needed.
- Refer caregiver(s) to an occupational therapist and/or lactation specialist to support normal feeding skills.

Infants with inborn errors of metabolism are treated according to established protocol (3).

Hyperglycemia

When blood glucose is 120 to 180 mg/dL (6.7 to 10 mM/L) during PN, consider reducing dextrose infusion by 1.5 to 3 g/kg/d (1 to 2 mg/kg/min). Consider providing insulin when blood glucose is markedly elevated (> 180 mg/dL or > 10 mM/L) or when dose of dextrose needed to maintain euglycemia is < 6 mg/kg/min **(C)**.

Recommendations for insulin infusion to treat hyperglycemia during PN are documented in the literature **(B)** (14,15).

Hypocalcemia

Symptomatic hypocalcemia requires provision of parenteral calcium gluconate, preferably as a continuous infusion, with meticulous attention to catheter integrity to prevent tissue damage due to extravasation. It is necessary to maintain normal serum levels of magnesium in order to sustain normal serum calcium levels **(C)** (1,2).

If vitamin D deficiency is suspected, provide 300 to 400 IU/d of vitamin D as cholecalciferol or ergocalciferol (1,2). Calcitriol may be needed, along with calcium supplements, in infants with permanent hypoparathyroidism (2).

Hypercalcemia

Reducing calcium intake and providing adequate hydration may be useful in treating hypercalcemia. However, primary hyperparathyroidism requires parathyroidectomy to normalize calcium metabolism. Preoperatively, restrict calcium intake. Postoperatively, the diet may require supplementation to achieve normal serum levels of calcium and vitamin D (2).

REFERENCES

1. Peters CJ, Hindmarsh PC. Management of neonatal endocrinopathies--Best practice guidelines. *Early Hum Dev.* 2007;83:553–561.
2. Sisto PAP. Endocrine disorders in the neonate. *Pediatr Clin North Am.* 2004;51:1141–1168.
3. Acosta P, Yannicelli S. *The Ross Metabolic Formula System: Nutrition Support Protocols.* 4th ed. Columbus, OH: Ross Products Division/Abbott Laboratories; 2001.
4. Harris DL, Weston PH, Harding JE. Incidence of neonatal hypoglycemia in babies identified as at risk. *J Pediatr.* 2012;161:787–791.
5. Adamkin D and Committee on Fetus and Newborn. Clinical report: postnatal glucose homeostasis in late-preterm and term infants. *Pediatr.* 2001;575–579.
6. Chapter 32. Hypoglycemia in infants and children. Kleinman RE, Greer FR, eds. *Pediatric Nutrition.* Elk Grove Village, IL: American Academy of Pediatrics 2014;771–789.
7. Kao LS, Morris BH, Lally KP, Stewart CD, Huseby V, Kennedy KA. Hyperglycemia and morbidity and mortality in extremely low birth weight infants. *J Perinatol.* 2006;26:730–736.
8. Hays SP, Smith EO, Sunehag AL. Hyperglycemia is a risk factor for early death and morbidity in extremely low birth-weight infants. *Pediatr.* 2006;118:1811–1818.
9. Kalhan S, Kilic I. Carbohydrate as nutrient in the infant and child: range of acceptable intake. *Eur J Clin Nutr.* 1999;53:S94–S100.
10. Hay Jr WW, Brown LD, Denne SC. In Koletzko B, Poindexter B, Uauy R, eds. Energy requirements, protein-energy metabolism and balance, and carbohydrates in preterm infants. *Nutritional Care of Preterm Infants: Scientific Basis and Practical Guidelines*. Basel, Switzerland: Karger; 2014;64–81. *World Review of Nutrition and Dietetics*. vol 110.
11. Hooy SK, Amorde-Spalding K. Infants of diabetic mothers. In: Groh-Wargo S, Thompson M, Cox JH, eds. *Nutritional Care for High-Risk Newborns.* 3rd ed. Chicago, IL: Precept Press; 2000:535–546.
12. Cowett RM. The infant of the diabetic mother. In: Hay WW. *Neonatal Nutrition and Infant Metabolism.* St Louis, MO: Mosby Year Book; 1991:419–431.

13. Bromiker R, Rachamim A, Hammerman et al. Immature sucking patterns in infants of mothers with diabetes. *J Pediatr*. 2006;149:640–3.
14. Thabet F, Bourgeois J, Guy B, Putet G. Continuous insulin infusion in hyperglycaemic very-low-birth-weight infants receiving parenteral nutrition. *Clin Nutr.* 2003;22:545–547.
15. Ng SM, May JE, Emmerson AJ. Continuous insulin infusion in hyperglycaemic extremely-low-birth-weight neonates. *Biol Neonate*. 2005;87:269–272.

Chapter 15

Osteopenia of Prematurity

Michelle Johnson, RD, CSP, LD

DISEASE STATE

Osteopenia of prematurity is defined as reduced bone mass of infants who were born before or during maximal inutero mineral accretion—80% of which occurs in the third trimester (1). Incidence is estimated to be 23% in very low birth weight (VLBW) infants and 55% in extremely low birth weight (ELBW) infants (2).

Osteopenia of prematurity is clinically silent. Biochemical monitoring should commence at 4 to 5 weeks postnatal age for infants with birth weight < 1,500 g. Alkaline phosphatase levels > 800 to 1,000 IU/L should be followed by radiographic evaluation of the wrist or knee and nutrition should be optimized. Serum phosphorus levels ≤ 4 mg/dL should prompt consideration of phosphorus supplementation and close monitoring of serum phosphorus (3).

Risk Factors (3)

- Preterm birth (< 27 weeks' gestational age [GA])
- VLBW (< 1,500 g)
- Prolonged PN (> 4 to 5 weeks)
- Enteral feedings with low mineral content/bioavailability: unfortified human milk, infant formulas with

mineral levels designed for term infants, soy-based infant formulas

- Chronic use of medications that increase mineral excretion (eg, diuretics, steroids)
- Low activity levels (lack of mechanical stimulation of muscles and bones)
- Severe chronic lung disease (CLD) with use of loop diuretics and fluid restriction
- Chronic history of necrotizing enterocolitis (NEC)

PREVENTIVE NUTRITION

The goal is to match intrauterine bone mineral accretion rates by optimizing energy, protein, general nutrient intakes (for bone matrix formation), and mineral intake (for mineralization of the matrix) (4). Enteral nutrition (EN) is preferred over parenteral nutrition (PN) for providing recommended mineral intake.

Optimize calcium and phosphorus intakes in PN. Recommendations include 65 to 100 mg/kg/d of calcium and 50 to 80 mg/kg/d of phosphorus in a ratio of 1 to 1.5:1 by weight (mg Ca:mg Phos) **(C)** (5). Strategies to assist with optimization include at least 2.5 g/kg/d of amino acid in 120 to 150 mL/kg/d; add cysteine to decrease the pH of the PN solution, which allows for greater solubility of calcium and phosphorus; and consult a clinical pharmacist to individualize and maximize calcium and phosphorus using solubility curves **(C)** (4).

To improve mineral stores, initiate minimal enteral nutrition (MEN), commonly 15 to 20 mL/kg/d, as soon as cardiorespiratory stability is achieved **(C)** (6,7).

Compared with the use of unfortified human milk or term formula, human milk supplemented with commercially available multinutrient human milk fortifier (HMF) or a preterm formula results in compositional weight gain and bone mineral content more similar to the reference fetus **(A)** (4). See Table 15.1 (3,5) for select enteral nutrient intake recommendations.

Limit use of mineral-depleting medications when feasible.

Table 15.1 Enteral Nutrient Intake Recommendations

Nutrient	Enteral Recommendation	Reference
Calcium	120–200 mg/kg per day	5
Phosphorus	60–140 mg/kg per day	5
Calcium:Phosphorus ratio (by weight)	1.5–1.7:1	3
Vitamin D	200 to 400 IU/d	3

Source: Data are from references 3 and 5.

TREATMENT NUTRITION

Wean from PN if possible. If not, maximize calcium and phosphorus in PN **(C)** (8). Start MEN if possible, and advance to or continue fortified human milk or preterm formula. If fortified human milk feedings or preterm formula feedings are not tolerated or not medically indicated for longer than 1 week, supplement feedings with 20 mg/kg/d of elemental calcium and 10 to 20 mg/kg/d of elemental phosphorus. Increase gradually to maximums of 70 to 80 mg/kg/d of elemental calcium and 40 to 50 mg/kg/d of elemental phosphorus. Select supplements based on availability, osmolality, mineral bioavailability, and fluid limitations. Provide calcium and phosphorus supplements separately to improve absorption. Avoid use of steroids and loop diuretics. Advise caregivers to handle infant cautiously to minimize risk of fractures. Evaluate for presence of cholestasis and vitamin D adequacy. Monitor serum phosphorus and serum alkaline phosphatase levels every 1 to 2 weeks, and monitor radiographs every 5 to 6 weeks until radiographic evidence of osteopenia is resolved **(C)** (3).

Although physical activity programs to promote weight gain and bone mineralization are not routinely recommended at this time, meta-analysis of 4 small studies revealed a positive effect of a passive range of motion program on daily weight gain and linear growth **(B)** (9).

CONTINUING CARE

VLBW infants discharged from the neonatal intensive care unit (NICU) at a period of rapid growth may still be at risk for osteopenia, particularly if breastfed without fortification or if fed term formula. For infants with osteopenia or who are at high risk for development of osteopenia after discharge, human milk fortifiers or preterm formulas historically used only in the hospital could be continued for approximately 12 weeks postdischarge **(C)** (10). Postdischarge follow-up should include evaluation of growth, laboratory indices, nutrient intake, and feeding regimen.

REFERENCES

1. Demarini S. Calcium and phosphorus nutrition in preterm infants. *Acta Paediatr.* 2005;94(Suppl 449):S87–S92.
2. Taylor SN, Hollis BW, Wagner CL. Vitamin D needs of preterm infants. *NeoReviews*. 2009;10:e590–e599.
3. Abrams SA. Committee on nutrition. Calcium and vitamin D requirements of enterally fed preterm infants. *Peds*. 2013;131:e1676–e1683.

4. American Academy of Pediatrics, Committee on Nutrition. Nutritional needs of the preterm infant. In: Kleinman RE, Greer FR, eds. *Pediatric Nutrition.* 7th ed. Elk Grove Village, IL: American Academy of Pediatrics; 2014:83–121.
5. Mimouni FB, Mandel D, Lubetzky R, Senterre T. In Koletzko B, Poindexter B, Uauy R, eds. Calcium, phosphorus, magnesium and vitamin D requirements of the preterm infant. *Nutritional Care of Preterm Infants: Scientific Basis and Practical Guidelines*. Basel, Switzerland: Karger; 2014:140–151. *World Review of Nutrition and Dietetics*. vol 110.
6. Kelly A, Kovatch KJ, Garber SJ. Metabolic bone disease screening practices among U.S. neonatologists. *Clin Peds*. 2014;53:1077–1083.
7. Ramani M, Ambalavanan N. Feeding practices and necrotizing enterocolitis. *Clin Perinatol*. 2013;40:1–10.
8. Figueras-Aloy J, Álvarez-Domínguez E, Pérez-Fernández JM, Moretones-Suñol G, Vidal-Sicart S, Botet-Mussons F. Metabolic bone disease and bone mineral density in very preterm infants. *J Pediatr.* 2014;164(3):499–504.
9. Schulzke SM, Kaempfen S, Trachsel D, Patole SK. Physical activity programs for promoting bone mineralization and growth in preterm infants. *Cochrane Database Syst Rev* 2014;4. CD005387. doi:10.1002/14651858.CD005387.pub3.
10. Groh-Wargo S, Thompson M. Managing the human-milk–fed, preterm, VLBW infant at NICU discharge. *ICAN: Infant, Child, & Adolescent Nutrition*. 2014;6:262–269.

Chapter 16

Neonatal Abstinence Syndrome

Marsha Dumm, MS, RD, LD

DISEASE STATE

Neonatal abstinence syndrome (NAS) is a constellation of symptoms seen in newborn infants withdrawing from maternal drug use. The recent increased incidence of NAS is well documented and represents significant healthcare costs related to treatment of withdrawal and increased length of hospital stay (1). Both licit and illicit maternal drug use are problematic: infants are more likely to be preterm, be born small for gestational age, have longer hospital stays, and experience feeding problems (2). Infants diagnosed with NAS are at higher risk of intrauterine growth restriction (IUGR) due to a hostile maternal environment at the time of conception as well as nutrient inadequacy during the pregnancy, and these patients will present a challenge to the neonatal dietitian (3).

Symptoms of NAS usually appear within 24 to 72 hours of birth, depending on the type of narcotic, and may be exacerbated by maternal tobacco use, multidrug exposure, and disruption of the mother-infant relationship (4). Preterm infants may exhibit fewer or less severe symptoms than term infants due to a shorter duration of exposure (5). Symptoms include high-pitched crying and inconsolable agitation as well as respiratory distress, yawning, sneezing, fever, mottled skin, gastrointestinal dysfunction, and excessive sucking (6,7). Gastrointestinal dysfunction manifests as frequent and severe diarrhea with perianal excoriation. Excessive sucking and hyperphagia are frequently seen; however, excessive weight gain does not necessarily accompany this feeding pattern and it may be necessary to concentrate formula to 22 or 24 kilocalories per fluid ounce to support growth.

PREVENTIVE NUTRITION

NAS cannot be prevented by nutrition; however, fetal growth restriction is less likely with a pregnant woman who is in treatment since she is less likely to suffer nutritional inadequacies.

TREATMENT NUTRITION

Mother's own milk is preferred for all infants but can be especially important in the management of NAS. Mothers in treatment with methadone or buprenorphine should be encouraged to provide milk (8). Opioid-exposed infants who are breastfed have shorter hospital stays and are less likely to require pharmacologic treatment (9,10). Mothers who are HIV positive or using illicit drugs or alcohol should not provide milk. Achieving normal postnatal growth is the goal for infants in treatment for NAS. Increasing nutrient density of formula feedings and human milk may be required. While there is no supporting evidence, low lactose and soy formulas have become popular for treatment of the temporary lactase deficiency caused by diarrhea during withdrawal.

ADDITIONAL (NONNUTRITION) TREATMENT OPTIONS

Morphine, methadone, and phenobarbital are used to control symptoms of withdrawal. Standardized scoring may be used to evaluate the infant's symptoms and response to narcotic doses (7). Narcotic dose is decreased when scores are stable and symptoms have diminished. While there is no recognized standard for treatment of these infants, a recent study suggests that adherence to formalized weaning protocol may reduce the length of hospital stay (11). Infants with low withdrawal scores, as well as those receiving tapering narcotic treatment, may benefit from nonpharmacologic treatment. Nursing strategies to minimize infant symptoms include decreasing external stimulation, soft lighting, and swaddling (5).

REFERENCES

1. Patrick SW, Shumacher RE, Benneyworth BD, Krans EE, McAllister JM, Davis MM. Neonatal abstinence syndrome and associated health care expenditures. United States 2000–2009. *JAMA*. 2012;307(18):1934–1940.
2. Creanga AA, Sabel JC, Ko JY, Wasserman CR, Shapiro-Mendoza CK, Taylor P, Barfield W, Cawthon L, Paulozzi LJ. Maternal drug use and its effect on neonates: a population-based study in Washington state. *Obstet Gynecol*. 2012;119(5):924–933.
3. Prada JA, Tsang RC. Biological mechanisms of environmentally induced causes of intrauterine growth retardation. *Eur J Clin Nutr*. 1998;52(Suppl 1):S1–S7.
4. Hodgson ZG, Abrahams RR. A rooming-in program to mitigate the need to treat for opiate withdrawal in the newborn. *J Obstet Gynaecol Can*. 2002;34(5):475–481.
5. Kaltenback K, Berghella, Finnegan L. Opioid dependence during pregnancy. Effects and management. *Obstet Gynecol Clin North Am*. 1998;25(1):139–151.

6. Behnke M, Smith VC; Committee on Substance Abuse; Committee on Fetus and Newborn. Prenatal substance abuse: short- and long-term effects on the exposed fetus. *Pediatrics*. 2013;131:e1009–e1024. http://pediatrics.aappublications.org/content/131/3/e1009.full. Accessed May 6, 2015.
7. Finnegan LP, Connaughton JF Jr, Kron RE, Emich JP. Neonatal abstinence syndrome: assessment and management. *Addict Dis*. 1975;2(1–2):141–158.
8. Kocherlakota P. Neonatal abstinence syndrome. *Pediatrics*. 2014;134(2):e547–e561.
9. Brown M, Hayes M, LaBrie S. Breast feeding is associated with decreased risk and length of treatment for neonatal abstinence syndrome (NAS) in methadone and buprenorphine exposed infants. Poster presented at Pediatric Academic Societies and Asian Society for Pediatric Research. Joint Meeting 2011. Boston, MA.
10. McQueen KA, Murphy-Oikonen J, Gerlach K, Montelpare W. The impact of infant feeding method on neonatal abstinence scores of methadone-exposed infants. *Adv Neonatal Care*. 2011;11(4):282–290.
11. Hall ES, Wexelblatt SL, Crowley M, Grow JL, Jasin LR, Klebanoff MA, McClead RE, Meinzen-Derr J, Mohan VK, Stein H, Walsh MC; OCHNAS Consortium. A multicenter cohort study of treatments and hospital outcomes in neonatal abstinence syndrome. *Pediatrics*. 2014;134(2):e527–e534.

Chapter 17

Discharge and Follow-up

Sharon Groh-Wargo, PhD, RD, LD

OBJECTIVES

- Recognize appropriate growth following NICU discharge.
- Provide appropriate nutrition treatment plans for both breast- and bottle-fed infants to support recovery postdischarge.
- Identify appropriate vitamin and mineral supplement regimens at discharge and during follow up.

INTRODUCTION

Increasing numbers of preterm, very low birth weight (VLBW) infants survive to discharge from the hospital (1). The goal of nutrition management is for the discharged preterm infant to achieve the body composition and rate of growth of a term infant of the same postconceptional age, although opinion and practice vary on how to achieve this (2–7). This chapter outlines nutritional management principles for prematurely born infants at discharge and during follow-up.

CORRECTED AGE

Chronological age (or "postnatal age") is the time (in days, weeks, months, etc.) elapsed since birth. This is different from "postmenstrual age," which is gestational age (GA) plus chronological age. Corrected age, defined as age from estimated term birth, is preferred to the term *adjusted age* and is used in nutritional assessment of infants born prematurely (8). For example:

- GA of 27 weeks when born on May 1: 13 weeks before estimated term date of August 1, (40 weeks – 27 weeks = 13 weeks, or 3 months' preterm)
- Chronological age of 6 months on November 1: 26 weeks past actual date of birth
- Corrected age of 3 months on November 1: 13 weeks past expected term date of birth (26 weeks – 13 weeks = 13 weeks, or 3 months)

Corrected age is used for preterm infants for at least the first year and up to 3 years but often, in practice, until 2 years, when the transition from the World Health Organization (WHO) to the Centers for Disease Control (CDC) growth charts is made (8).

DISCHARGE CRITERIA

Criteria for discharge readiness is focused on achievement of developmental milestones rather than attainment of a specific weight and include (9):

- Respiratory stability—usually in room air but sometimes on oxygen by nasal cannula, free of apnea and bradycardia; with a tracheostomy in rare cases

- Ability to take sufficient enteral feedings—usually by breast and/or bottle; by nasogastric tube, gastrostomy tube, or intravenously in selected cases
- Maintenance of normal body temperature outside the isolette
- Availability of an appropriate home environment and prepared caregivers
- Scheduled appointments for home visits, developmental follow-up clinic, well-child care, and with the Supplemental Nutrition Program for Women, Infants and Children (WIC)

NUTRITION ASSESSMENT

Nutrition follow-up of the infant discharged from the neonatal intensive care unit (NICU) is recommended (9). The registered dietitian assesses growth, interprets laboratory results, reviews feeding tolerance, performs qualitative or quantitative intake analysis, and offers anticipatory guidance.

Growth Assessment

Infants born during the third trimester of pregnancy are expected to gain approximately 17 to 21 g/kg/d in weight, until they reach > 2 kg; then gains of 30 to 35 g/d are expected (10). Growth of ≥ 0.9 cm/week is expected in length and head circumference (see Chapter 1, Nutrition Assessment). After reaching a corrected age of 40 weeks, growth velocity should approximate term infants, as shown in Table 17.1 (11).

Table 17.1 Velocity of Weight and Length Gain After Term

Age, months	Weight, g/d Mean (3rd–97th Percentile Range)		Length, cm/wk Mean (3rd–97th Percentile Range)	
	Males	Females	Males	Females
Up to 2	36 (22–52)	31 (19–46)	1.0 (0.7–1.2)	0.9 (0.7–1.1)
2–4	24 (13–35)	22 (12–33)	0.6 (0.4–0.8)	0.6 (0.4–0.8)
4–6	15 (7–26)	14 (6–24)	0.4 (0.2–0.6)	0.4 (0.2–0.6)
6–9	10 (4–19)	10 (4–18)	0.3 (0.2–0.5)	0.3 (0.2–0.5)
9–12	8 (2–16)	8 (1–15)	0.3 (0.1–0.4)	0.3 (0.1–0.4)
12–18	9 (2–12)	7 (2–13)	0.3 (0.1–0.4)	0.3 (0.2–0.4)
18–24	6 (2–11)	6 (2–12)	0.2 (0.1–0.3)	0.2 (0.1–0.3)

Source: Data are from reference 11.

Some infants, especially extremely low birth weight (ELBW) infants, approach NICU discharge with anthropometric measurements below birth percentiles (12). This growth pattern is labeled extrauterine growth restriction (EUGR) if parameters plot below the 10th percentile. To recover from EUGR, a period of catch-up growth is required. Catch-up growth occurs when the velocity of weight gain is higher than that expected for age. Achievement of catch-up growth is not well defined. Anthropometric measurements that plot above the 5th to 10th percentile on a growth chart for term infants may be considered adequate catch-up by some. Others want growth to retrack along the birth percentiles before declaring the achievement of catch-up growth. Still others expect a downward resetting of the growth trajectory (13). The rate at which catch-up growth should occur is also controversial. Excessive rates of weight gain in early infancy have been associated with adverse long-term metabolic outcomes; however, one noted expert states, "While slow growth . . . has some benefits for later cardiovascular outcome, it risks under-nutrition and its adverse consequences, and has a profound adverse effect on later cognition. Currently, the balance of risks favors the brain and preterm infants should be fed with specialized products to support rapid growth (at least at the intrauterine rate)" (14).

Growth charts are used to visually monitor progress, and an excellent online tool is available to assist in growth assessment (PediTools; www.peditools.org). Table 17.2 compares characteristics of charts commonly used at discharge and during follow-up from the NICU (10,11,15–18).

Table 17.2 Comparison of Selected Growth Charts

Chart (Reference)	Considerations
Fenton, 2013 (10)	• Range from 22–50 weeks: 22–40 (cross-sectional intrauterine growth) plus 40–50 weeks (postnatal term reference [WHO]) • Separate male and female charts • Frequent choice at NICU discharge and immediate follow-up • Growth chart located at http://ucalgary.ca/fenton/2013chart
Olsen, 2010 (15)	• Range from 23 to 41 weeks (based on cross-sectional intrauterine growth data from a US population) • Separate male and female charts
Infant Health and Development Program, 1996, 1997 (16,17)	• Longitudinal data of preterm infants 32 weeks' gestational age to 38 months; only charts available to compare growth to a group of preterm infants • Use with caution; measurements plot higher than when compared with term longitudinal data, possibly leading to a false impression that growth is adequate

(continued)

Table 17.2 Comparison of Selected Growth Charts (continued)

Centers for Disease Control and Prevention (CDC), 2000 (18)	• US data, birth to 20 years • Graphs start at term corrected age • Recommended for children ≥ 2 years • Growth chart located at www.cdc.gov/growthcharts/cdc_charts.htm
World Health Organization (WHO), 2006 (11)	• Worldwide standard, birth to 5 years • Infant growth based on predominantly or exclusively human milk feeding • Graphs start at term corrected age • Recommended for term to 2 years of age • Growth chart located at www.who.int/childgrowth/en/

Source: Data are from references 10, 11, and 15–18.

Laboratory Assessment

The frequency of laboratory assessment decreases after discharge and is individualized to each patient's condition. Table 17.3 lists some common conditions requiring continued surveillance.

Table 17.3 Laboratory Surveillance After Hospital Discharge

Parameter	Indication(s)
Phosphorus, alkaline phosphatase, 25(OH)D	Osteopenia
Liver function tests including direct bilirubin	Cholestasis
Complete blood count	Anemia; screening for iron deficiency at 9–12 months' corrected age
Albumin, prealbumin	Poor nutrition history, slow growth, edema

Feeding Tolerance

Prematurely born infants are at increased risk for poor feeding and growth failure, especially those with neurologic deficits, developmental delay, or sensory impairment. Physical, cognitive, motor, neurologic, visual, and auditory assessments offer insight into feeding abilities (9). Common problems include vomiting, constipation, and poor feeding.

Vomiting

Some minor spitting up is expected in young infants. However, vomiting that is projectile, substantial, and occurring after most feedings or resulting in poor growth is not normal. Possible causes are overfeeding, improper mixing of formula, uncontrolled reflux, or bowel stricture/obstruction (especially following necrotizing enterocolitis). Conservative treatment includes anticipatory guidance regarding feeding schedules and normal infant response to feeding, as well as education about formula preparation.

Constipation

Constipation is defined as pebble-like, hard stools two or fewer times per week. Constipation is rare in infants fed human milk. On average (19,20):

- Breastfed infants 0 to 3 months have 3 yellow stools per day.
- Formula-fed infants 0 to 3 months have 2 yellow, brown, or green stools per day.
- Infants 6 to 12 months have 1 to 2 stools per day.

Possible causes of constipation include improper mixing of formula, milk protein allergy, developmental delay/neurologic disease, and adverse effects of medication.

Prune, pear, or apple juice full-strength or diluted 1:1 with water (starting with 1 to 2 teaspoons/d for infants < 5 kg and up to 1 to 2 oz/d for larger infants), or a stool softener such as lactulose (1 to 3 mL/kg 1 or 2 times per day) are possible treatments for constipation (19,21).

Poor Feeding

Vague descriptions of poor feeding or refusal to eat are often reported by caregivers of former VLBW infants. Possible causes include fatigue in the recovering preterm infant, poor oxygenation in the infant with cardiorespiratory disease, a chaotic home environment, constipation, neurologic disease, and infection. Feeding specialists, such as occupational and speech therapists, can develop individualized treatment plans to improve the feeding skills of the caregivers and the endurance of the baby. Schedules with defined limits to feeding sessions (usually ≤ 30 minutes per feeding) and daily goals for amounts of milk and/or solids can be helpful (22).

Intake Assessment

Nutrient intake recommendations are available for VLBW infants at ages and weights common at discharge (6,7,23–25). Table 17.4 compares selected values (6,7,23,24). The recommendations assume no accumulated nutrient deficits. Babies who are able to go home but have anthropometric and/or laboratory assessments that suggest marginal sufficiency, deficiency, and/or EUGR may need greater nutrient intake.

Table 17.4 Nutrient Intake Recommendations for VLBW Infants at NICU Discharge (per kg/d)

	Energy (kcal)	Protein (g)	PE Ratio (g/100 kcal)	Ca (mg)	P (mg)
Lapillonne, et al (2013;2014) (6,7)[a]	115–127	2.5–3.1	2.2–2.4	70–140	35–90
Rigo and Senterre (2006) (23)[b]	116–123	2.8–3.2	2.4–2.6		
Rigo and Senterre ("with need of catch-up growth") (2006) (23)[b]	115–121	3–3.4	2.6–2.8		
Ziegler (24)[c]	131	3.4	2.6		

Abbreviations: VLBW, very low birth weight; NICU, neonatal intensive care unit; PE, protein to energy

[a]For 34–38 weeks in-hospital and at discharge for babies without risk factors and/or no accumulated nutritional deficits

[b]For 36–40 weeks

[c]For body weight 1,800–2,200 g assuming no accumulated nutrient deficits

Source: Data are from references 6, 7, 23, and 24. Reprinted from Groh-Wargo S and Thompson M. Managing the human-milk-fed, preterm, VLBW infant at NICU discharge: The sprinkles dilemma. *Infant, Child & Adolescent Nutrition*. 2014;6(5):262–269, with permission of Sage.

Assessment of enteral intake is quantitative or qualitative based on anthropometric data.

- Qualitative if growth is adequate: *what* is fed; general feeding schedule
- Quantitative if growth falters: *what* and *how much* is fed; details of feeding schedule; calculation of estimated energy intake and other nutrients as appropriate

Although there is no universally accepted convention, a gradual transition from intake recommendations for preterm infants to the Dietary Reference Intakes (DRIs) is made based on either attainment of term-corrected age and/or catch-up in weight on an appropriate growth chart. Daily energy and protein recommendations for infants past term are available as Adequate Intakes (AIs) and have been set using estimated intakes of human milk (26). (See Tables 3.2–3.5 for complete lists of infant AIs.) Reference body weights are available for the two age categories in infancy. Estimated daily energy (mean kcal ± 2 standard deviations) and protein (g) AIs are as follows:

- Birth to 6 months (6 kg): 90 (72 to 108) kcal/kg and 1.5 g protein/kg
- 7 to 12 months (9 kg): 80 (64 to 96) kcal/kg and 1.2 g protein/kg

AIs should be used cautiously, in conjunction with growth assessment, in preterm infants.

BREASTFEEDING AND HUMAN MILK

Human milk is the preferred feeding for all infants. Hospitalization and prematurity complicates the newborn breastfeeding period because (*a*) separation requires the mother to pump and frequently leads to diminished milk supply, and (*b*) prematurity of 1 month or more requires tube feeding in the hospital and a period of transition to the breast that often includes some bottle feeding. Many preterm infants cannot, or will not be able to, breastfeed exclusively at the time of discharge. Preterm infants exclusively fed human milk are known to have slower growth than preterm infants fed preterm or enriched formula, but they benefit from enhanced development and protection against infection (27,28).

Nutrition Goals

Nutrition goals for the breastfeeding mother and her baby at discharge are as follows:

- Promote adequate weight gain, including necessary catch-up growth.
- Ensure good nutritional status of protein, calcium, phosphorus, and other micronutrients.
- Maintain or build breast milk supply.
- Sustain or improve feedings at the breast.
- Limit bottle and formula feeding to that required for the first and second goals.

Goals are individualized based on the condition of the baby at discharge, the supply of breast milk, and the wishes of the mother. Box 17.1 suggests management options for six common scenarios at discharge (29).

Box 17.1 Nutrition Management Option for Human Milk–Fed VLBW Infants at NICU Discharge: Six Mother-Baby Situations

1. No longer pumping with no stored EBM
- Baby with risk factors[a]: PF24; transition to PTDF at 3.5 kg
- Baby without risk factors: PTDF

2. No longer pumping but with significant stored EBM
- Baby with risk factors[a]: FHM for several weeks with transition to PTDF when stores of EBM exhausted
- Baby without risk factors: HM alternated with PTDF with transition to PTDF when stores of EBM exhausted

3. Still pumping with little or no stored EBM, mother interested in feeding the baby at the breast
- Baby with risk factors[a]: PFHP24 from bottle alternated with direct BF; transition to PTDF at 3.5 kg; lactation support to get baby to the breast; continue pumping
- Baby without risk factors: PTDF from bottle alternated with direct BF; lactation support to get baby to the breast; continue pumping

(continued)

Box 17.1 Nutrition Management Option for Human Milk–Fed VLBW Infants at NICU Discharge: Six Mother-Baby Situations (continued)

4. Still pumping with little or no stored EBM, mother not interested in feeding the baby at the breast

- Baby with risk factors[a]: PFHP24 alternated with EBM from bottle; transition to PTDF at 3.5 kg; continue pumping 8–10 times/day to improve supply
- Baby without risk factors: PTDF alternated with EBM from bottle; continue pumping 8–10 times/day to improve supply

5. Still pumping with significant stored EBM, mother interested in feeding the baby at the breast

- Baby with risk factors[a]: FHM from bottle for ≥ ½ of the feedings until 3.5 kg, then BF:PTDF in 3:1 ratio; lactation support to move from pumping to breastfeeding
- Baby without risk factors: 60–90 mL/d PF30 "booster" (divided) fed along with HM until 3.5 kg then plain HM; lactation support to move from pumping to breastfeeding

6. Still pumping with significant stored EBM, mother not interested in feeding the baby at the breast

- Baby with risk factors[a]: FHM from bottle for ≥ ½ of the feedings until 3.5 kg, then HM alternated with PTDF; continue pumping
- Baby without risk factors: 60–90 mL/d PF30 "booster" (divided) fed along with HM until 3.5 kg, then plain HM; continue pumping

Abbreviations: EBM: expressed breast milk; BF: breastfeeding; PTDF: preterm discharge formula (eg, Similac NeoSure, Enfamil EnfaCare); FHM: fortified human milk (commercial human milk fortifier 1 packet to 25 mL EBM); PF24: preterm formula 24 kcal/oz (eg, Similac Special Care, Enfamil Premature, Gerber Good Start Premature); PFHP24: preterm formula high-protein 24 kcal/oz (eg, Similac Special Care High Protein, Enfamil Premature High Protein, Gerber Good Start Premature High Protein); PF30: preterm formula 30 kcal/oz (eg, Similac Special Care 30, Enfamil Premature 30, Gerber Good Start Premature 30); HM: human milk; BW: birth weight.

[a]Risk factors/accumulated nutritional deficits: Anthropometric: ≤ 1,250 g BW and ≤ 2 kg at discharge, ≤ 2 kg at discharge with any BW; history of weight gain < 25g per day the week before discharge. Gestational age: ≤ 28 weeks at birth, ≤ 37 weeks at discharge. Biochemical: Alkaline phosphatase ≥ 600 IU/L, serum phosphorus ≤ 6 mg/dl, BUN ≤ 9 mg/dl. Nutritional: Total parenteral nutrition ≥ 4 weeks; volume restriction < 120 mL/kg per day;

Box 17.1 Nutrition Management Option for Human Milk–Fed VLBW Infants at NICU Discharge: Six Mother-Baby Situations (continued)

history of use of low nutrient density, tolerance, and/or term formulas (eg, soy, protein hydrolysate, or amino acid–based formulas), or unfortified human milk. Miscellaneous: Radiological evidence of bone demineralization and/or fracture(s); chronic use of mineral-wasting medications (ie, furosemide).

Source: Reprinted from Groh-Wargo S, and Thompson M. Managing the human-milk-fed, preterm, VLBW infant at NICU discharge: The sprinkles dilemma. *ICAN: Infant, Child, & Adolescent Nutrition*. 2014;6(5):262–269. Adapted with permission of Sage.

Fortification, Enrichment, and Supplementation of Human Milk at Discharge

Continued fortification of expressed human milk using a commercial human milk fortifier (HMF) may be indicated at discharge, would be safe for infants < 3.5 kg or who are taking less than full volume of fully fortified (1:25) milk, and could be appropriate for infants who have significant risk factors such as (29):

- Anthropometric (≤ 1,250 g birth weight [BW] and ≤ 2 kg at discharge; ≤ 2 kg at discharge with any BW; history of weight gain < 25 g/d the week before discharge; EUGR infant still requiring catch-up growth)
- GA (≤ 28 weeks at birth; ≤ 37 weeks at discharge)
- Biochemical (alkaline phosphatase ≥ 600 U/L, serum phosphorus ≤ 6 mg/dL; blood urea nitrogen [BUN] ≤ 9 mg/dL)
- Nutritional (total parenteral nutrition [TPN] ≥ 4 weeks; volume restriction < 120 mL/kg per day; history of low nutrient density, term and/or tolerance formula [eg, soy, protein hydrolysate, or amino acid–based], or unfortified human milk)
- Miscellaneous (radiological evidence of bone demineralization and/or fracture[s]; chronic use of mineral-wasting medications)

ELBW and very sick infants are the most likely to fall into this category (29). In a randomized clinical trial, VLBW infants who were fed human milk fortified with a commercial HMF (1 packet to 25 mL expressed human milk) for half of their feedings for 12 weeks following discharge had improved nutrient intake, growth, body composition, and visual acuity compared with similar babies fed human milk alone (30–32). Regarding feeding the preterm infant after discharge, the American Association of Pediatrics (AAP) recommends that "strong consideration should be given to fortification of human milk for a minimum of 12 weeks for those infants who weigh less than 1,250 g at birth and/or have incurred intrauterine or extrauterine growth restriction, because they represent the highest nutritional risk categories" (5).

Enrichment of expressed human milk using a preterm discharge formula (PTDF) powder is a common practice for infants who need energy-dense feedings. Soy, protein hydrolysate, and amino acid–based formulas are not recommended for preterm infants, but enrichment of expressed human milk with these formulas is sometimes chosen to increase the caloric density of feedings for infants who do not tolerate milk-based products such as HMF or PTDF. None of these enrichment options meet the protein or micronutrient requirements of VLBW infants. The AAP specifically recommends against feeding soy formula to preterm infants (33).

Table 17.5 (6,25,34,35) compares the intake of selected nutrients with recommendations for preterm infants provided by the following:

- Exclusive human milk
- Human milk enriched with PTDF
- Human milk alternated with PTDF, fortified human milk (FHM), or preterm formula high-protein 24 kcal/oz (PFHP24)

- Human milk followed by "nutrition boosters"
- Fortified human milk

Table 17.5 Comparison of Intake for Selected Nutrients (per kg/d) from Human Milk–Based Feeding Options for VLBW Infants at NICU Discharge: 2 kg Infant Receiving ~120 kcal/kg per day

Feeding Type (kcal/oz)	mL/kg	g/kg protein	Mg/kg Ca	Mg/kg P	Mcg/kg Zn
HM (20)	180	1.6	40	23	360
Enriched HM (24)[a]	150	1.9	55	32	513
HM alternated with PTDF (21)	170	2.6	91	52	910
HM alternated with FHM (22)	165	2.6	122	69	1050
HM alternated with PFHP24 (22)	165	3	132	70	1129
HM plus 60–120 ml PF30 "booster"[b]	165	2.1–2.8	84–132	48–74	726–1,123
FHM (24)	150	3.4	188	106	1,610
Nutritional Recommendations	135–200	2.5–3.1[c]	70–140[c]	35–90[c]	1,100–2,000

Abbreviations: HM: human milk; Enriched HM: human milk with added preterm-discharge formula powder to make ~24 kcal/oz (estimated using an average of the 2 commercially available preterm-discharge formulas) (so-called "sprinkles"); PTDF: preterm discharge formula (eg, Similac NeoSure, Enfamil EnfaCare); FHM: fortified human milk (commercial human milk fortifier 1 packet to 25 mL EBM) (estimated using an average of the two commercially available concentrated liquid human milk fortifiers); PFHP24: preterm formula high protein 24 kcal/oz (eg, Similac Special Care HP, Enfamil Premature HP, Gerber Good Start Premature HP); PF30: preterm formula 30 kcal/oz (eg, Similac Special Care 30, Enfamil Premature 30, Gerber Good Start Premature 30)

(continued)

Table 17.5 Comparison of Intake for Selected Nutrients (per kg/d) from Human Milk–Based Feeding Options for VLBW Infants at NICU Discharge: 2 kg Infant Receiving ~120 kcal/kg per day (continued)

Note: Shading indicates intakes that do not meet recommendations.
[a] "Sprinkles"
[b]As amount of "booster" increases, volume contribution from human milk decreases (34).
[c]Assuming no accumulated nutrient deficits
Source: Data are from references 6, 25, 34, and 35. Reprinted from Groh-Wargo S, Thompson M. Managing the human-milk-fed, preterm, VLBW infant at NICU discharge: The sprinkles dilemma. *ICAN: Infant, Child, & Adolescent Nutrition.* 2014;6(5):262–269, with permission of Sage.

The various intakes increase in nutrient density from top to bottom in the table. Neither human milk alone nor human milk enriched with PTDF meet the needs of the VLBW infant at discharge. Human milk alternated with various preterm formulas or with FHM provides an intake within the range of nutritional recommendations. Continued full fortification of human milk may be indicated in specific situations, as outlined in Box 17.1, and would generally be limited to ELBW preterm infants who remain < 3.5 kg at discharge (29). HMFs are available with a doctor's prescription through some state WIC programs and on selected private insurance policies. They are not widely available, however, which complicates the discharge planning for babies who need them.

Summary: Breastfeeding and Human Milk at Discharge

Most mothers of preterm infants can be persuaded to pump and are able to successfully provide milk for their babies during the acute phase of care, but will need help in the transition from tube and/or bottle feeding if they want to breastfeed. Special attention to protein and minerals ensures adequate nutrition. Continued fortification with a commercial HMF or supplementation with a preterm formula is considered for the highest-risk preterm babies. Larger preterm babies may benefit from supplementation with a PTDF.

FORMULA CHOICES

If breastfeeding is not chosen or is stopped before 1 year corrected age, and expressed human milk is not available, infants are fed a commercial infant formula. Most preterm infants receiving preterm formula in the NICU are transitioned to PTDF in preparation for hospital discharge. Somewhat larger preterm or late preterm infants may receive PTDF as their initial feeding and go home on the same formula. Although some controversy exists about the efficacy of PTDF to improve growth and outcomes for preterm infants, the AAP and the European Society of Pediatric Gastroenterology, Hepatology and Nutrition (ESPGHAN), many noted experts, and most clinical trials support their use after NICU discharge (3,5–7,14,36–40). The duration of PTDF use is usually inversely related to birth weight; the smallest babies receive the formulas for the longest time (38,39). Continued feeding of preterm formula at discharge may be indicated for infants who have significant anthropometric, gestational age, biochemical, nutritional, or other risk factors similar to those described for infants that are considered for continued human milk fortification at discharge (36). Soy, protein hydrolysate, and amino acid–based formulas may be needed for infants who do not tolerate milk-based products such as preterm formula or PTDF. These alternative formulas needed for intolerance are not intended for preterm infants, may be inadequate in protein and some micronutrients, and require vitamin/mineral supplementation. Box 17.2 (2,3,5,33,36–41) reviews issues to consider for formula-fed prematurely born infants at discharge.

Box 17.2 Infant Formula Choices for Prematurely Born Infants at Discharge

Preterm[a]

- **Examples**: Gerber Good Start Premature[b]; Enfamil Premature[c]; Similac Special Care[d]
- **Availability**: Individual ready-to-feed bottles in 20- and 24-kcal/oz strengths
- **Likely choice for**: Infants < 1,250 g at birth who have ongoing nutritional risk factors at discharge
- **Duration of use**: 3.5 kg weight or 500 mL/d is approximate upper limit for safe use due to high concentration of fat-soluble vitamins in preterm formula; transition to PTDF when upper limits reached
- **Evidence**: When fed in the early postdischarge period, facilitates faster nutritional repletion than standard formula (36)

Preterm Discharge[a]

- **Examples**: Enfamil EnfaCare[c]; Similac NeoSure[d]
- **Availability**: Ready-to-feed and powder; usual concentration of 22 kcal/oz but reconstitution of powder can be individualized; iron-fortified
- **Likely choice for**: Infants born, or ready for discharge, at approximately 1.8 kg
- **Duration of use**: Recommendations vary: Individualized to optimize growth trajectory over first year of life (5); until 40–52 weeks' postconceptional age (3); consider longer use for ELBW infants, especially if preterm formula stopped before term corrected age
- **Evidence**: May promote better weight, length and head circumference gain, and improved fat-free mass and bone mineral content, especially in infants < 1,250 g at birth, although this is controversial (2,3,5,33,36–40)

(continued)

Box 17.2 Infant Formula Choices for Prematurely Born Infants at Discharge (continued)

Other[a]

- **Examples**: Soy, protein hydrolysate, and amino acid–based formulas (various brand names)
- **Availability**: Powders, liquid concentrates, and/or ready-to-feed; usually iron-fortified
- **Likely choice for**: Infants intolerant to the intact protein in preterm or PTDF
- **Duration of use**: Until 1 year corrected age
- **Evidence**: Last choice; inadequate levels of some micronutrients, especially calcium, phosphorus, and zinc (33,41)

Abbreviations: PTDF, preterm discharge formula; ELBW, extremely low birth weight

[a]Refer to Tables 3.1 and 3.2 in Chapter 3 for more detailed formula information.

[b]Nestle, Vevey, Switzerland

[c]Mead Johnson, Evansville, IN

[d]Abbott Nutrition, Columbus, OH

Source: Data are from references 2, 3, 5, 33, and 36–41.

Safety Issues

To ensure safety when feeding formula:

- The US Food and Drug Administration recommends mixing infant formula "using ordinary cold tap water that's brought to a boil and then boiled for one minute and cooled" (42). For most infants older than 3 months' corrected age, water no longer needs to be boiled and formula prepared with water directly from the tap is satisfactory (43).
- Due to the risk of contamination from the bacterium *Cronobacter sakasakii* (formerly known as *Enterobacter sakasakii*) (44), powdered formula is handled with care. Safe handling practices include mixing the smallest batch practical so that storage time is limited to fewer than 24 hours.

- All mixing and measuring equipment and all bottles and nipples are thoroughly cleaned and air-dried before use.
- All caregivers are given thorough mixing and measuring instructions prior to discharge. Techniques are periodically reviewed after discharge.
- Bottled and spring water are not sterile unless labeled as such.
- Use of the microwave for warming infant formula is strongly discouraged.
- Formula left in the bottle at the end of a feeding is discarded (no longer than 60 minutes after the beginning of the feed).
- Product expiration dates are noted and expired formula discarded.
- Once powdered formula is opened, it should be discarded after 30 days.

SUPPLEMENTS

Vitamin and/or mineral supplements may be indicated for some preterm infants at discharge. Box 17.3 lists common feeding regimens at discharge, micronutrients that will likely fall below recommendations for preterm infants, and suggested infant vitamin/mineral supplements (3,5–7,45–47). Vitamin D recommendations are based on a goal of 400 IU per day (45). In the first 6 months, recommended iron intakes are 2 to 4 mg/kg/d (preterm) and 1 mg/kg/d (term) (5,46).

Box 17.3 Suggested Vitamin and Mineral Supplements at Discharge for a 2-kg Infant Consuming Various Feeding Regimens

Exclusive human milk (HM) or enriched HM (HM mixed with PTDF powder to ~24 kcal/oz)

Micronutrient considerations:

- All water- and fat-soluble vitamins
- Most minerals, including calcium, phosphorus, and zinc; begin source of iron by 1 month
- Begin fluoride after 6 months if there is no source of fluoridated water

Suggested supplements[a]*:*

- AquADEKs 1 mL[b] QD until full term size (about 3.4 kg), then 400 IU vitamin D as Tri-vi-sol[c] or D-only drop 1 ml QD until taking 1 qt per day of formula
- Iron by 1 month at 2–4 mg/kg QD until 1 year
- Fluoride, as appropriate, 0.25 mg QD

HM alternated with PTF, PTDF, FHM [1 packet/vial:25 mL HM], or half-strength FHM [1 packet/vial:50 mL HM]

Micronutrient considerations:

- Since products vary and the amount of formula supplement will vary—check total micronutrient intake to assess need for vitamin supplement
- Begin source of iron by 1 month
- Begin fluoride after 6 months corrected age if there is no source of fluoridated water

Suggested supplements[a]*:*

- Poly-vi-sol[c] 1 mL QD until infant is full term size, then 400 IU vitamin D as Tri-vi-sol[c] or D-only drop 1 mL QD until taking 1 qt/d of formula
- Iron by 1 month at 2–4 mg/kg QD until 1 year
- Fluoride, as appropriate, 0.25 mg QD

(continued)

Box 17.3 Suggested Vitamin and Mineral Supplements at Discharge for a 2-kg Infant Consuming Various Feeding Regimens (continued)

FHM [1 packet/vial:25 mL HM]

Micronutrient considerations:

- Iron if HMF does not contain iron or infant needs more than provided in HMF; *Caution:* do not use after infant reaches 3.5 kg or intake of 500 mL QD as excessive nutrient intake may occur

Suggested supplement[a]*:* By 1 month, iron 2–4 mg/kg

PTF 20/24 kcal/oz with iron

Micronutrient considerations:

- Iron if infant needs more than provided by formula; *Caution:* do not use after infant reaches 3.5 kg or intake of 500 mL QD as excessive nutrient intake may occur

Suggested supplement[a]*:* By 1 month, iron 2–4 mg/kg

PTDF 22 kcal/oz with iron

Micronutrient considerations:

- Vitamin supplement may be required if < 2 kg because total volume of intake will be relatively small
- Iron if infant needs more than provided by formula
- Begin fluoride after 6 months if there is no source of fluoridated water

Suggested supplements[a]*:*

- Poly-vi-sol[c] 1 mL until infant is full term size, then 400 IU vitamin D as Tri-vi-sol[c] or D-only drop 1 ml QD until taking 1 qt per day of formula
- Iron by 1 month at 2–4 mg/kg QD until 1 year;
- Fluoride, as appropriate, 0.25 mg QD

(continued)

Box 17.3 Suggested Vitamin and Mineral Supplements at Discharge for a 2-kg Infant Consuming Various Feeding Regimens (continued)

Soy, protein hydrolysate, or amino acid based–formula with iron

Note: These formulas are not intended for preterm infants.

Micronutrient considerations:

- Products vary; supplement may be required for many vitamins and minerals especially if total intake volume is relatively small
- Iron if infant needs > 2 mg/kg/d provided by iron-fortified formula
- Begin fluoride after 6 months if there is no source of fluoridated water

Suggested supplements[a]*:*

- Poly-vi-sol[c] 1 mL until infant is full term size then 400 IU vitamin D as Tri-vi-sol[c] or D-only drop 1 mL QD until taking 1 qt per day of formula
- Iron by 1 month at 2–4 mg/kg QD until 1 year
- Fluoride, as appropriate, 0.25 mg QD

Abbreviations: HM, human milk; FHM, fortified human milk; PTF, preterm formula; PTDF, preterm discharge formula; HMF, human milk fortifier; QD, every day

[a]All suggested times are corrected age.

[b]AquADEKs (Yasoo Health Inc., Johnson City, TN) contains zinc, substantial vitamin A (87% as beta carotene), but no calcium or phosphorus; consider additional mineral supplementation if osteopenia exists.

[c]Mead Johnson, Evansville, IN

Source: Data are from product handbooks and references 3, 5–7, and 45–47.

When the infant reaches full-term size (approximately 3.4 kg) and makes the transition to the DRIs, the need for supplements greatly decreases, assuming all problems of prematurity, such as osteopenia, have resolved. The need for vitamin D supplementation remains for older preterm infants who are exclusively breastfed or who receive less than 1 quart per day of a commercial infant formula

(45,48). Iron drops are given to exclusively human milk–fed infants or to formula-fed infants who need more than the 2 mg/kg/d provided by most commercial, iron-fortified infant formulas. A source of iron is needed no later than 1 month corrected age for preterm infants and 4 months of age for late preterm or term infants (5,46). After 6 months' corrected age, an intake for preterm and term infants of 2 mg/kg/d and 11 mg/d of iron, respectively, is needed (5,46). Additionally, a daily supplement of 0.25 mg of fluoride is recommended for infants who are exclusively breastfed, are considerably volume-restricted, or who receive either ready-to-feed formula or formula reconstituted with nonfluoridated water (47). The fluoride supplement is given as a single nutrient supplement.

FEEDING PROGRESSION

Anticipatory guidance about feeding progression is offered to all caregivers at discharge and when the infant is seen in follow-up. Corrected age and developmental assessment is used to determine readiness for advancement. An overview of the first year follows (43,49):

- Human milk/breastfeeding or infant formula provides the primary source of nutrition for the entire first year.
- Solid foods are introduced from a spoon at approximately 4 to 6 months' corrected age; new foods are introduced no faster than approximately one every 5 days.
- Solid foods with more texture (Stages 2 and 3), finger foods, and cup feeding are introduced after 6 months' corrected age.
- Cow's milk is delayed until 12 months corrected age.

Common problematic feeding behaviors include resistance of new flavors/textures; picky eating; and constant nibbling, snacking and/or sipping from bottle—often called "cruising" or "grazing." Ineffective responses to problematic feeding behaviors include forced feeding, persistent/constant coaxing, and offering rewards for eating. Many helpful suggestions for health care professionals caring for preterm infants at home can be found at the Gaining and Growing: Assuring Nutritional Care of Preterm Infants website (http://staff.washington.edu/growing).

SUMMARY

High-risk newborns deserve careful nutrition assessment at discharge and close follow-up after discharge to ensure optimal growth and development. In conclusion:

- Use corrected age for nutritional assessment and recommendations.
- Calculate velocity of weight and length gain and compare with that expected for age.
- Plot serial anthropometric measurements on an appropriate growth chart.
- Evaluate quality of dietary intake for all infants. Quantitative analysis is indicated for infants with growth failure.
- Encourage breastfeeding and/or continued use of expressed human milk, but evaluate nutritional adequacy. Consider continued fortification or supplementation with a nutrient-dense preterm formula for the smallest infants until term age or size.
- For formula-fed infants, recommend PTDF. Consider continued preterm formula for the smallest infants until term age or size.

- Monitor intake of all micronutrients, especially vitamin D, calcium, phosphorus, zinc, and iron, and assure adequate intake.
- Anticipate difficulty with feeding transitions, especially for the smallest babies and those with continuing medical/surgical problems.
- Offer anticipatory nutrition guidance to caregivers.

REFERENCES

1. Fanaroff AA, Stoll BJ, Wright LL, Carlo WA, Ehrenkranz RA, Stark AR, Bauer CR, Donovan EF, Korones SB, Laptook AR, Lemons JA, Oh W, Papile LA, Shankaran S, Stevenson DK, Tyson JE, Poole WK, NICHD Neonatal Research Network. Trends in neonatal morbidity and mortality for very low birthweight infants. *Am J Obstet Gynecol*. 2007;196(2);147.e1–e8.
2. Greer FR. Post-discharge nutrition: what does the evidence support? *Semin Perinatol.* 2007;31:89–95.
3. ESPGHAN Committee on Nutrition. Feeding preterm infants after hospital discharge. *J Pediatr Gastroenterol Nutr.* 2006;42:596–603.
4. Nzegwu NI, Ehrenkranz RA. Post-discharge nutrition and the VLBW infant: To supplement of not supplement? *Clin Perinatol*. 2014;41:463–474.
5. American Academy of Pediatrics, Committee on Nutrition. Nutritional needs of the preterm infant. In Kleinman RE, Greer FR, eds. *Pediatric Nutrition.* 7th ed. Elk Grove Village, IL: American Academy of Pediatrics; 2014:83–121.
6. Lapillonne A, O'Connor DL, Wang D, Rigo R. Nutritional recommendations of the late-preterm infant and the preterm infant after hospital discharge. *J Pediatr*. 2013;162:S90–S100.
7. Lapillonne A. In Koletzko B, Poindexter B, Uauy R, eds. Feeding the Preterm Infant after Discharge. *Nutritional Care of Preterm Infants: Scientific Basis and Practical Guidelines*. Basel, Switzerland: Karger; 2014:264–277. *World Review of Nutrition and Dietetics*. vol. 110.
8. Committee on Fetus and Newborn, AAP. Age terminology during the perinatal period. *Pediatrics.* 2004;114:1362–1364.
9. Committee on Fetus and Newborn, AAP. Hospital discharge of the high-risk neonate. *Pediatrics*. 2008;122:1119–1126.

10. Fenton TR, Kim JR. A systematic review and meta-analysis to revise the Fenton growth chart for preterm infants. *BMC Pediatrics*. 2013;13:59. www.biomedcentral.com/1471-2431/13/59. Accessed March 17, 2015.
11. World Health Organization. The WHO Child Growth Standards. 2006. www.who.int/childgrowth/en. Accessed November 18, 2014.
12. Ehrenkranz RA, Younes N, Lemons JA, Fanaroff AA, Donovan EF, Wright LL, Katsikiotis V, Tyson JE. Oh W, Shankaran S, Bauer CR, Korones SB, Stoll BJ, Stevenson DK, Papile L. Longitudinal growth of hospitalized very low birth weight infants. *Pediatrics.* 1999;104:280–289.
13. Cole TJ, Statnikov Y, Santhakumaran S, Pan H, Modi N, on behalf of the Neonatal Data Analysis Unit and the Preterm Growth Investigator Group. Birth weight and longitudinal growth in infants born below 32 weeks' gestation: a UK population study. *Arch Dis Child Fetal Neonatal Ed.* 2014;99:F34–F40.
14. Lucas A. Long-term programming effects of early nutrition – implications for the preterm infant. *J Perinatol.* 2005;25:S2–S6.
15. Olsen IE, Groveman SA, Lawson ML, Clark RH, Zemel BS. New intrauterine growth curves based on United States data. *Pediatrics.* 2010;125:e214–e224.
16. Guo SS, Wholihan K, Roche AF et al. 1996. Weight-for-length reference data for preterm, low birthweight infants. *Arch Pediatr Adolesc Med.* 150;964–970.
17. Guo SS, Roche AF, Chumlea WC, Casey PH, Moore WM. Growth in weight, recumbent length, and head circumference for preterm low-birthweight infants during the first three years of life using gestation-adjusted ages. *Early Hum Dev.* 1997;47:305–325.
18. Kuczmarski RJ, Ogden CL, Grummer-Strawn LM, Flegal KM, Guo SS, Wei R, Mei Z, Curtin LR, Roche AF, Johnson CL. CDC growth charts: United States. *Adv Data.* 2000;(314):1–27.
19. Baker SS, Liptak GS, Colletti RB, Croffie JM, Lorenzo CD, Ector W, Nurko S. Evaluation and treatment of constipation in children: Summary of the updated recommendations of the North American Society of Pediatric Gastroenterology, Hepatology and Nutrition. *J Pediatr Gastroenterol Nutr.* 2006;43:405–407.
20. Malacaman EE, Abbousy FK, Crooke D, Nauyok G. Effect of protein source and iron content of infant formula on stool characteristics. *J Pediatr Gastroenterol Nutr.* 1985;4:771–773.

21. Benninga MA, Voskuijl WP, Taminiau JAJM. Childhood constipation: is there new light in the tunnel? *J Pediatr Gastroenterol Nutr*. 2004;39:448–464.
22. Klein MD, Delaney TA, eds. *Feeding and Nutrition for the Child with Special Needs.* San Antonio, TX: Therapy Skill Builders; 1994.
23. Rigo J, Senterre J. Nutritional needs of premature infants: current issues. *J Pediatr* 2006;149:S80–S88.
24. Ziegler EE. Protein requirements of very low birth weight infants. *J Pediatr Gastroenterol Nutr.* 2007;45:S170–S174.
25. Agostoni C, Buonocore G, Carnielli VP, De Curtis M, Darmaun D, Decsi T, Domellöf M, Embleton ND, Fusch C, Genzel-Boroviczeny O, Goulet O, Kalhan SC, Kolacek S, Koletzko B, Lapillonne A, Mihatsch W, Moreno L, Neu J, Poindexter B, Puntis J, Putet G, Rigo J, Riskin A, Salle B, Sauer P, Shamir R, Szajewska H, Thureen P, Turck D, van Goudoever JB, Ziegler EE; ESPGHAN Committee on Nutrition. Enteral nutrient supply for preterm infants: commentary from the European Society of Paediatric Gastroenterology, Hepatology and Nutrition Committee on Nutrition. *J Pediatr Gastroenterol Nutr.* 2010;50:85–91.
26. Institute of Medicine. *Dietary Reference Intakes: Energy, Carbohydrate, Fiber, Fat, Fatty Acids, Cholesterol, Protein, and Amino Acids.* Washington, DC: National Academy Press; 2002/2005. www.nal.usda.gov/fnic/DRI/DRI_Energy/energy_full_report.pdf (Accessed November 18, 2014)
27. Schanler RJ, Shulman RJ, Lau C. Feeding strategies for premature infants: beneficial outcomes of feeding fortified human milk versus preterm formula. *Pediatrics.* 1999;103:1150–1157.
28. O'Connor DL, Jacobs J, Hall R, Adamkin D, Auestad N, Castillo M, Connor WE, Connor SL, Fitzgerald K, Groh-Wargo S, Hartmann EE, Janowsky J, Lucas A, Margeson D, Mena P, Neuringer M, Ross G, Singer L, Stephenson T, Szabo J, Zemon V. Growth and development of premature infants fed predominantly human milk, predominantly premature infant formula, or a combination of human milk and premature formula. *J Pediatr Gastroenterol Nutr.* 2003;37:437–446.
29. Groh-Wargo S, Thompson M, 2014. Managing the human-milk-fed, preterm, VLBW infant at NICU discharge: The sprinkles dilemma. *ICAN: Infant, Child, & Adolescent Nutrition.* 2014;6(5):262–269.

30. O'Connor DL, Khan S, Weishuhn K, Vaughan J, Jefferies A, Campbell DM, Asztalos E, Feldman M, Rovet J, Westall C, Whyte H; Postdischarge Feeding Study Group. Growth and nutrient intakes of human milk-fed preterm infants provided with extra energy and nutrients after hospital discharge. *Pediatrics.* 2008;121:766–776.
31. Aimone A, Rovet J, Ward W, Jefferies A, Campbell DM, Asztalos E, Feldman M, Vaughan J, Westall C, Whyte H, O'Connor DL; Post-Discharge Feeding Study Group. Growth and body composition of human milk-fed premature infants provided with extra energy and nutrients early after hospital discharge: 1-year follow-up. *J Pediatr Gastroenterol Nutr.* 2009;49(4):456–466.
32. O'Connor DL, Weishuhn K, Rovet J, , Mirabella G, Jefferies A, Campbell DM, Asztalos E, Feldman M, Whyte H, Westall C; Post-Discharge Feeding Study Group. Visual development of human milk-fed preterm infants provided with extra energy and nutrients after hospital discharge. *JPEN J Parenter Enteral Nutr.* 2012;36:349–353.
33. Bhatia J, Greer F; Committee on Nutrition. Use of soy protein-based formulas in infant feeding. *Pediatrics.* 2008;121:1062–1068.
34. University of California San Diego, Health System, Support Premature Infant Nutrition (SPIN). http://health.ucsd.edu/specialties/obgyn/maternity/newborn/nicu/spin/Pages/default.aspx. Accessed March 17, 2015.
35. American Academy of Pediatrics, Committee on Nutrition. Nutritional needs of the preterm infant. In Kleinman RE, Greer FR, eds. *Pediatric Nutrition.* 7th ed. Elk Grove Village, IL: American Academy of Pediatrics; 2014:1431–1432. Accessed November 18, 2014.
36. Young L, Morgan J, McCormick FM, McGuire W. Nutrient-enriched formula versus standard term formula for preterm infants following hospital discharge. *Cochrane Database Syst Rev.* 2012;(3). doi: 10.1002/14651858.CD004696.pub4. www.nichd.nih.gov/cochrane_data/mcguirew_13/mcguirew_13.html. Accessed March 17, 2015.
37. Brunton JA, Saigal S, Atkinson SA. Growth and body composition in infants with bronchopulmonary dysplasia up to 3 months corrected age: a randomized trial of a high-energy nutrient-enriched formula fed after hospital discharge. *J Pediatr.* 1998;133:340–345.

38. Carver JD, Wu PYK, Hall RT, Ziegler EE, Sosa R, Jacobs J, Baggs G, Auestad N, Lloyd B. Growth of preterm infants fed nutrient-enriched or term formula after hospital discharge. *Pediatrics.* 2001;107:683–689.
39. Lucas A, Fewtrell MS, Morley R, Singhal A, Abbott RA, Isaacs E, Stephenson T, MacFadyen UM, Clements H. Randomized trial of nutrient-enriched formula versus standard formula for postdischarge preterm infants. *Pediatrics.* 2001;108:703–711.
40. Koo WWK, Hockman EM. Posthospital discharge feeding for preterm infants: effects of standard compared with enriched milk formula on growth, bone mass, and body composition. *Am J Clin Nutr.* 2006;84:1357–1364.
41. Mithatsch WA, Franz AR, Hogel J, Pohlandt F. Hydrolyzed protein accelerates feeding advancement in very low birth weight infants. *Pediatrics.* 2002;110:1199–1203.
42. US Food and Drug Administration. FDA takes final step on infant formula protections. www.fda.gov/forconsumers/consumerupdates/ucm048694.htm. Accessed November 18, 2014.
43. Dietz WH, Stern L, eds. *American Academy of Pediatrics Guide to Your Child's Nutrition.* New York, NY: Villard; 1999.
44. Centers for Disease Control and Prevention. *Enterobacter sakazakii* infections associated with the use of powdered infant formula--Tennessee, 2001. *MMWR Morb Mortal Wkly Rep.* 2002;51:297–300.
45. Wagner CL, Greer FR and the Section on Breastfeeding and Committee on Nutrition, American Academy of Pediatrics. Clinical Report – Prevention of rickets and vitamin D deficiency in infants, children, and adolescents. *Pediatrics.* 2008;122:1142–1152.
46. Baker RD, Greer FR and the Committee on Nutrition, American Academy of Pediatrics. Clinical report – Diagnosis and prevention of iron deficiency and iron-deficiency anemia in infants and young children (0–3 years of age). *Pediatrics.* 2010;126:1040–1050.
47. American Academy of Pediatrics, Committee on Nutrition. Fluoride supplementation for children: interim policy recommendations. *Pediatrics.* 1995;95:777.
48. American Academy of Pediatrics, Section on Breastfeeding. Breastfeeding and the use of human milk. *Pediatrics.* 2012;129:e827–e841.
49. Sullivan SA, Birch LL. Infant dietary experience and acceptance of solid foods. *Pediatrics.* 1994;93:271–277.

Appendix A

Nutrition Care Process

Janice Hovasi Cox, MS, RD, CSP

The Academy of Nutrition and Dietetics has developed a system for documenting nutrition care using standardized language to describe assessment, identify specific nutrition diagnoses, describe intervention, and identify measures to monitor and evaluate progress toward meeting the goals of intervention. This Nutrition Care Process (NCP) system supports and promotes individualized nutrition care by providing a framework for standardizing the process and the way in which this process is communicated. This process encourages critical thinking and supports the efficient and equitable provision of safe and effective nutrition care (1–4).

STEP 1: NUTRITION ASSESSMENT

For neonates, nutrition assessment begins with determining gestational age and *z* score or percentile ranking for anthropometric measurement, then comparing subsequent growth against established standards and obtaining relevant data from intake records, including parenteral, enteral, and oral nutrient intake. Other factors considered in nutrition assessment include biochemical data, medical tests, and procedures; physical examination findings, including feeding tolerance descriptions, presence and appearance of emesis, and description of stool characteristics; and client history information, such as family history of food allergy, intent to breastfeed, parental height, financial eligibility for supplemental food programs, and reading ability of parents or other caregivers. Accurate interpretations of these data yield assessments that lead to nutrition diagnoses and effective interventions.

STEP 2: NUTRITION DIAGNOSIS

Nutrition diagnosis is not a restatement of the medical diagnosis but the identification and specific labeling of the nutrition problem that the neonatal dietitian is responsible for treating. The nutrition diagnosis is defined by a statement that includes the following:

- Problem (P) or label that describes an alteration in nutritional status
- Etiology of the problem (E) or the cause or contributing factors that sustain the problem, and
- Signs and symptoms (S) that identify, characterize, or define the nutrition problem

For example, the medical diagnosis may be osteopenia of prematurity, but the nutrition diagnosis may be: "Inadequate vitamin intake, specifically vitamin D, and inadequate mineral intake, specifically calcium and phosphorus *(P),* related to increased nutrient needs and feeding intolerance associated with cow's milk protein–based human milk fortifier *(E),* as evidenced by serum phosphorus level less than 5.6 mg/dL and alkaline phosphatase level more than 900 U/L *(S).*"

STEP 3: NUTRITION INTERVENTION

Nutrition intervention involves specific actions to treat or resolve the nutrition problem. Intervention requires a change in one or more of the following:

- Food and nutrient delivery
- Nutrition education
- Nutrition counseling
- Coordination of nutrition care

The intervention is usually aimed at the etiology of the problem. For example, the nutrition intervention for a preterm infant with the nutrition diagnosis of inadequate vitamin D, calcium, and phosphorus intake might be to change nutrient delivery by the following nutrition prescription: "Provide standard dose of extensively hydrolyzed cow's milk protein–based human milk fortifier."

STEP 4: NUTRITION MONITORING AND EVALUATION

In the fourth NCP step, the success of the nutrition intervention may be measured as a change in the signs and symptoms of the problem, or by comparing specific indicators with established standards. For example, the patient with low serum phosphorus levels and elevated alkaline phosphatase may be monitored for changes in serum phosphorus levels. Serum alkaline phosphatase levels may remain elevated with increased osteoblastic activity, but serum phosphorus levels should become normal with adequate nutrient intake. By selecting the appropriate measure(s) of outcome, the neonatal dietitian can compare findings with the previous state, specific identified goals, and/or reference standards. The use of such standards to monitor and evaluate achievement of nutrition goals and resolution of the nutrition problem facilitates the assessment and comparability of outcomes and increases the validity and reliability of treatment modalities.

Standardized language has been developed for many of the parameters of nutrition assessment, diagnosis, intervention, monitoring, and evaluation. Publications that address the NCP and provide detailed lists and explanations of the standardized Nutrition Care Process Terminology are available through the Academy of Nutrition and Dietetics, and are included in the reference list (1–4).

Note: An online tool kit for the Nutrition Care Process as it is applied in the neonatal patient population is also available for purchase through the Academy of Nutrition and Dietetics (5).

REFERENCES

1. Lacey K, Pritchett E. Nutrition care process and model: ADA adopts road map to quality care and outcomes management. *J Am Diet Assoc.* 2003;103:1061–1072.
2. Academy of Nutrition and Dietetics. *eNCPT Nutrition Terminology Reference Manual: Dietetics Language for Nutrition Care.* 2014 ed. https://ncpt.webauthor.com. Accessed April 9, 2015.
3. Writing Group of the Nutrition Care Process/Standardized Language Committee. Nutrition care process and model part I: The 2008 update. *J Am Diet Assoc.* 2008;108:1113–1117.
4. Academy International Nutrition Care Process. http://aincp.webauthor.com. Accessed November 30, 2014.
5. American Dietetic Association. *Neonatal Nutrition Toolkit: A Practical Application of the Nutrition Care Process and Standardized Language to the NICU Setting.* Chicago, IL: American Dietetic Association; 2008.

Appendix B

Conversion Tables

Janice Hovasi Cox, MS, RD, CSP

ATOMIC WEIGHTS AND VALENCES

Element	Atomic Weight	Valence
Sodium	23	1
Potassium	39	1
Chloride	35	1[a]
Calcium	40	2
Phosphorus	31	3, 5
Magnesium	24	2

[a]Chloride may also have valences of 3, 5, and 7, but, for practical purposes, it has a valence of 1 for most nutritional compounds.

Equations

$$\frac{\text{mg} \times \text{Valence}}{\text{Atomic or molecular weight}} = \text{mEq}$$

$$\frac{\text{mEq} \times \text{Atomic or molecular weight}}{\text{Valence}} = \text{mg}$$

Atomic or molecular weight in mg = mM

mM × Atomic or molecular weight = mg

Sample Calculations

$$\frac{23 \text{ mg sodium} \times 1 \text{ (valence)}}{23 \text{ (atomic weight)}} = 1 \text{ mEq sodium}$$

$$\frac{24 \text{ mg magnesium} \times 2 \text{ (valence)}}{24 \text{ (atomic weight)}} = 2 \text{ mEq magnesium}$$

$$\frac{1 \text{ mEq calcium} \times 40 \text{ (atomic weight)}}{2 \text{ (valence)}} = 20 \text{ mg calcium}$$

$$\frac{31 \text{ mg phosphorus}}{31 \text{ (atomic weight)}} = 1 \text{ mM phosphorus}$$

$$1 \text{ mM potassium} \times 39 \text{ (atomic weight)} = 39 \text{ mg potassium}$$

Electrolytes and Minerals

Nutrient	Conventional Unit	Conversion Factor Multiply → ← Divide	SI Unit
Bicarbonate	mEq	1.0	mmol
Calcium	mEq	0.5	mmol
	mg	0.025	
Chloride	mEq	1.0	mmol
	mg	0.0282	
Copper	mcg	1.527	nmol
Magnesium	mEq	0.5	mmol
	mg	0.042	
Potassium	mEq	1.0	mmol
	mg	0.0256	
Phosphorus	mg	0.0323	mmol
Sodium	mEq	1.0	mmol
	mg	0.0435	mmol
Zinc	mcg	0.0153	μmol

Vitamins and Other Nutrients

Nutrient	Conventional Unit	Conversion Factor Multiply → ← Divide	SI Unit
Ascorbate (vitamin C)	mg	5.678	μmol
Biotin	ng	0.004093	nmol
Carotene (vitamin A)	mcg mcg	0.00186 1.667	μmol IU[a]
Carnitine	mg	6.25	μmol
Cholecalciferol (vitamin D-3)	ng mcg	0.002599 40.0	nmol IU[a]
25-OH-cholecalciferol	ng	0.002496	nmol
Choline chloride	mcg	7.163	mmol
Cyanocobalamin (vitamin B-12)	pg	0.0007378	pmol
Folic acid	ng	0.002266	nmol
Niacin (vitamin B-3)	mg	8.12347	μmol
Pantothenic acid	mcg	0.004562	μmol
Phylloquinone (vitamin K)	pg	2.22	nmol
Pyridoxine hydrochloride (vitamin B-6)	mg	4.8638	μmol
Retinol (vitamin A)	mcg mcg	0.003491 3.33	μmol IU[a]
Riboflavin (vitamin B-2)	mcg	2.657	nmol
Thiamin (vitamin B-1)	mcg	0.003324	μmol
Thiamin hydrochloride	mcg	0.002965	μmol
d-alpha tocopherol (vitamin E)	mg	2.322	μmol
d-alpha tocopherol	mg	1.49	IU[a]
d-alpha tocopheryl acetate	mg	1.36	IU
d-alpha tocopheryl acid succinate	mg	1.21	IU

(continued)

Nutrient	Conventional Unit	Conversion Factor Multiply → ← Divide	SI Unit
dl-alpha tocopherol	mg	1.0	IU
dl-alpha tocopheryl acetate	mg	1.0	IU
dl-alpha tocopheryl acid succinate	mg	0.89	IU
Triglycerides mg/dL	mg	0.00113	mmol

[a]Note on International Units (IU):
Vitamin A: 1 IU = 0.3μg retinol, 3.6 μg beta carotene, or 7.2 μg other vitamin A carotenoids
Vitamin D: 1 IU = 0.025 μg cholecalciferol
Vitamin E: 1 IU = 0.67 mg d-alpha-tocopherol, 0.74 mg d-alpha tocopheryl acetate, 0.83 mg d-alpha tocopheryl acid succinate, 1.12 mg dl-alpha tocopheryl acid succinate

NUTRIENT CONTENT PER GRAM OF COMPOUND

Compound (1 g)	Amount of Nutrient in Compound		
	mg	mEq	mM
Calcium (Ca)			
calcium chloride (27.3% Ca by wt)	273	13.6	6.8
calcium gluceptate (8.2% Ca by wt)	82	4.1	2.0
calcium gluconate (9.3% Ca by wt)	93	4.7	2.3
calcium carbonate (40% Ca by wt)	400	19.9	9.96
Chloride (Cl)			
calcium chloride (72.7% Cl by wt)	727	21	21
potassium chloride (47.7% Cl by wt)	477	13.6	13.6
sodium chloride (60.3% Cl by wt)	603	17.2	17.2
Copper (Cu) [a]			
copper chloride (37.4% Cu by wt)	374	—	—
copper sulfate (25.5% Cu by wt)	255	—	—

(continued)

Compound (1 g)	Amount of Nutrient in Compound		
	mg	mEq	mM
Magnesium (Mg)			
magnesium sulfate (20.2% Mg by wt)	202	16.8	8.4
Potassium (K)			
potassium acetate (39.8% K by wt)	398	10.2	10.2
potassium chloride (52.3% K by wt)	523	13.4	13.4
dibasic potassium phosphate (44.9% K by wt)	449	11.5	11.5
monobasic potassium phosphate (28.5% K by wt)	285	7.3	7.3
Phosphorus (P)			
di-/monobasic K phosphate (17.2% P by wt)	172	—	5.5
sodium phosphate (23.8% P by wt)	238	—	7.7
Sodium (Na)			
sodium acetate (17% Na by wt)	168	7.3	7.3
sodium bicarbonate (27.4% Na by wt)	274	11.9	11.9
sodium chloride (39.7% Na by wt)	397	17.2	17.2
sodium phosphate (31.2% Na by wt)	312	13.5	13.5
Zinc (Zn) [a]			
zinc chloride (47.8% Zn by wt)	478	—	—
zinc gluconate (14.3% Zn by wt)	143	—	—
zinc sulfate anhydrous (40.1% Zn by wt)	401	—	—
zinc sulfate heptahydrate (23% Zn by wt)	225	—	—

[a]Cu and Zn dosage ranges are in micrograms (mcg) per kilogram body weight if administered parenterally and < 10 mg/d enterally.

NUTRIENT CONTENT PER 1 ML OF SOLUTION

	Amount of Nutrient in Compound		
Compound (1 g)	**mg**	**mEq**	**mM**
Calcium			
calcium chloride 10% (1 g/10 mL)	27.3	1.4	0.7
calcium gluceptate 22% (1.1 g/5 mL)	18	0.9	0.4
calcium gluconate 10% (1 g/10 mL)	9.3	0.5	0.2
Chloride			
calcium chloride 10% (1 g/10 mL)	72.7	2.1	2.1
potassium chloride (14.8%)	70	2.0	2.0
sodium chloride (14.6%)	87.5	2.5	2.5
sodium chloride (23.4%)	140	4.0	4.0
Copper			
copper chloride (1.07 mg copper chloride)	0.4	—	—
copper sulfate (1.57 mg copper sulfate)	0.4	—	—
copper sulfate (7.85 mg copper sulfate)	2.0	—	—
Magnesium			
magnesium sulfate heptahydrate 10%	9.6	0.8	0.4
Phosphorus			
potassium phosphate	93	—	3.0
sodium phosphate	93	—	3.0
Potassium			
potassium acetate	39	1	1
potassium chloride 7.4% (0.74 g/10 mL)	39	1	1
potassium phosphate	172	4.4	4.4
Sodium			
sodium acetate 8.2%	23	1	1
sodium bicarbonate 4.2%	11.5	0.5	0.5
sodium bicarbonate 5%	13.8	0.6	0.6
sodium acetate 32.8%	92	4	4
sodium chloride 5.8%	23	1	1
sodium chloride 23.4%	92	4	4
Zinc			
zinc chloride (2.09 mg zinc chloride)	1	—	—
zinc sulfate (4.39 mg heptahydrate or 2.46 mg anhydrous)	1		
zinc sulfate (21.95 mg zinc sulfate)	5	—	—

Index

Page number followed by *t* indicates table, by *f* indicate figure, and by *b* box.

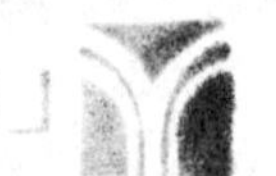

Libraries@Trocaire